RAW AWAKENING

LOSE **WEIGHT** | UNLEASH YOUR **ENERGY** | FEEL AND LOOK **SPECTACULAR**

RAW AWAKENING

YOUR ULTIMATE GUIDE TO THE **Raw Food Diet**

KRISTEN SUZANNE

CHRONICLE BOOKS
SAN FRANCISCO

Library of Congress Cataloging-in-Publication Data:
Suzanne, Kristen.
Raw Awakening : your ultimate guide to the raw food diet / Kristen Suzanne.
p. cm.
Includes index.
ISBN 978-1-4521-0649-6
1 Raw foods—Therapeutic use. I. Title.

TX740.S896 2012
613.2'65—dc23

2011036734

Manufactured in China

Designed by Allison Weiner
Typesetting by DC Typography
Cover photography by Leigh Beisch
Illustrations by Yuka Hollingsworth

10 9 8 7 6 5 4 3 2 1

Chronicle Books LLC
680 Second Street
San Francisco, California 94107
www.chroniclebooks.com

CONTENTS

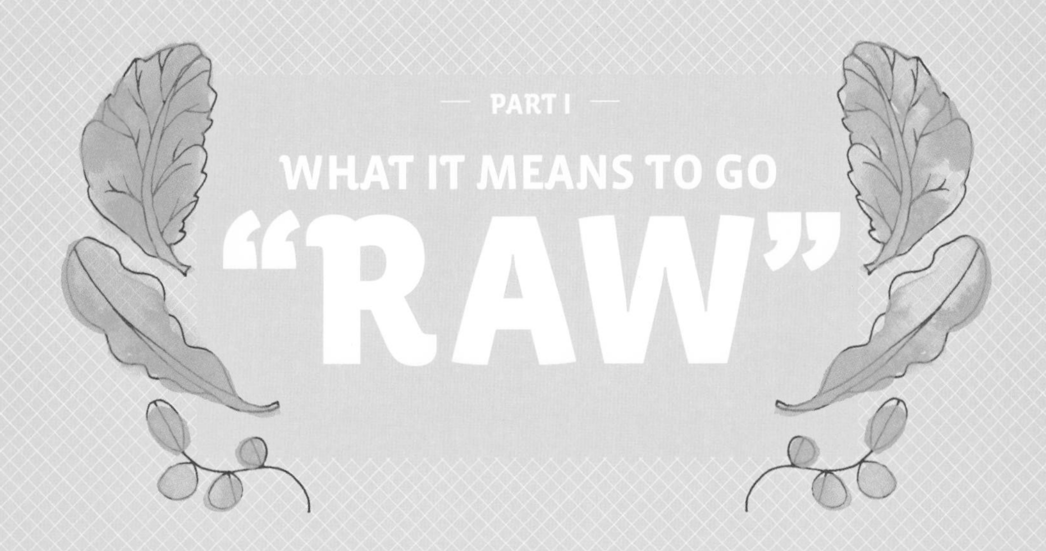

— PART I —

WHAT IT MEANS TO GO "RAW"

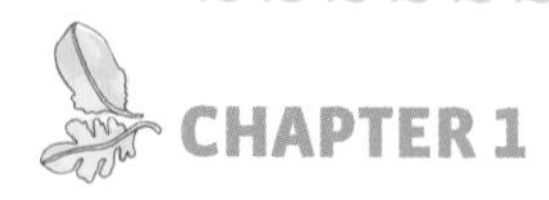

CHAPTER 1

WHY RAW?

Knowing is not enough; we must apply. Willing is not enough; we must do.
—Goethe

We've all heard time and again that we should eat more fruits and vegetables. The difference between that statement in the past versus today is that we now have exciting, delicious, and innovative ways to prepare fruits and vegetables, as evidenced by the skyrocketing popularity of "raw food," which has emerged as a completely new cuisine all its own. Eating raw no longer refers to fruit plates and a few boring sticks of carrot or celery. Among thousands of chefs, healthful-eating advocates, foodies, and ordinary people from all walks of life, "raw food" now refers to an exciting, energetic way of eating and living that is not only far more healthy than anything that's come before, but is also amazingly delicious and satisfying.

Eating "raw" refers to a diet of plant-based foods that are uncooked, minimally refined or processed, and very close to their natural state. Living a "raw food lifestyle" simply means that you try to make raw food a majority of what you eat. Some people start out with very little raw food in their diet; others dive in headfirst and seek to cut out nearly all cooked food at once. And there are many degrees in between; you don't have to eat 100 percent raw starting tomorrow, or ever, for that matter. To get started, anyone can enjoy noticeably improved health and vitality by switching to eating at least 50 percent raw foods (ideally, 100 percent plant-based).

While 50 percent might seem like a lot, it's actually very easy once you learn the basics. In fact, once you start seeing the results of including more fresh organic raw foods in your diet, you'll want more and more, because that's exactly what your body will tell you it wants. And once you taste gourmet raw dishes that you can make yourself, you'll wonder why you would ever want to eat cooked food at all!

When you eat raw food, especially gourmet raw food (which is very easy to make, as we'll discuss), the flavors "pop." They shock your palate and wake up your taste buds. You have an experience that goes to your core, like an awakening or an enlightenment. You'll feel so amazing after eating a raw meal that adding more and more raw food to your diet will feel like the natural thing to do. It will become a no-brainer for you, and very easy once you start adapting to the lifestyle. With raw food cuisine, your world is suddenly open to experiencing bold flavors, sensuous textures, and surprising new combinations of fresh fruits, vegetables, herbs, nuts, and seeds as you never imagined they could be—it's simply incredible!

Eating more raw plant-based food is one of the most amazing things you can do for yourself. I would even say that it's essential if you're looking to experience life at its fullest. The trick, then, is to find the most convenient and habitual ways to incorporate more raw food into your daily food choices. But don't worry; if you follow the principles outlined in this book, the raw lifestyle is actually very easy.

By simply eating more of the foods your body was designed to digest, and thereby getting rid of the junk that makes us unhealthy, you'll be able to do amazing things: lose unwanted weight, eliminate or reduce cellulite, improve digestion, experience restful sleep, gain incredible amounts of energy, have brighter eyes and younger-looking skin, experience mental clarity and energy as never before, and have a new lease on life—literally, owing to raw food's ability to prevent and even reverse some of the diseases that are the leading causes of death in the industrialized world.

When I'm eating raw, I am on top of the world. It's almost hard to describe, but I'll try! Sounds are more crisp, colors are more electric, and tastes are more vibrant. Everything is better. My skin is better. My sleep is better. My energy is better. My attitude is better. I feel empowered and unstoppable. Do you want to see what that's like for yourself? Do you want to feel better than you've ever felt in your life? Well, you can!

MY BACKGROUND

I've always had a passion for nutrition, athletics, and staying in shape. As a result, I found myself reading and trying every diet out there over a period of fifteen years. During this time, a friend introduced me to John Robbins' book *Diet for a New America*, which was the first time I learned about eating a plant-based diet. I was so enthralled, I blazed through the book in only a few sittings, and when I was done reading it, that was it: I was also done consuming animal products. Forever. It moved me that much. The book moves most people who read it, in fact. I remember reading it at a coffee shop and having more than one person come up to me to say that they too had read the book and that it had changed their life.

With my newfound enthusiasm for a plant-based, or vegan, diet (meaning no meat, fish, poultry, eggs, or dairy), I was on the hunt for recipes. And that is how I found raw. One day, I was in Whole Foods Market searching for a good cookbook with recipes that used lots of vegetables when I came upon a book about raw food. "Hmm . . . raw food?" I thought. On one hand, it sounded strange. But at the same time, something resonated deep inside me as I realized that, no, the way our culture eats nowadays is what's strange. Insane, even—it's killing us. And then we try to fight the diseases with drugs rather than fixing the problem where it started. Eating raw food is like personally rediscovering our roots and our place in the natural world. It strips away ten thousand years of bad habits.

No wonder, then, that the food tastes so—right. It's hard to explain, but when I'm eating raw food, I feel as though I'm digging down to a more primal place, replacing the foods that seemed "normal" to me simply because I was raised with them with the foods that were abundant on the earth when humanity first began. In fact, when I was flipping through that book in the store, just reading its recipes instantly struck a chord. They sounded so amazing that I bought the book, took it home, and read it voraciously in one night. A recipe book! Funny, right? But it's true—each page made me more excited about the idea of eating more raw food. I was enticed by the recipes loaded with fresh ingredients and the promises of high energy, glowing skin, and feeling amazing. I literally could not wait to get started!

The very next day, I started adding more raw foods to my diet, and I've never looked back.

WHAT DOES "RAW" MEAN?

What does "raw" really mean? In today's culinary vernacular, the term "raw food" refers to 100 percent plant-based food that has never been heated above 115° to 118°F (46° to 48°C), at which point proteins become damaged. Sometimes you'll hear the term *raw* used interchangeably with *living*. There is a small difference. Some "living foods," such as freshly picked fruit, are considered to be in a living state, where their enzymes are active and available. *Raw* can refer to foods that do not readily have their enzymes available, even though they have not been heated or destroyed. Nuts and seeds, for example, are considered "raw" (if they have not been heat treated), but they are not "living" because their enzyme inhibitors are intact. It's during the process of soaking nuts and seeds that their enzyme inhibitors are deactivated, converting them from merely raw into living food (more on that later). Some ingredients, like unpasteurized miso and tamari, are not considered raw because heat was used in the process of making them, but the products were later cultured with a beneficial bacterium, making them "living" foods.

WHY RAW?

There are many reasons to eat raw plant-based foods. My short answer to the question "Why raw?" is simple: It could change your life. It changed mine.

With fresh, pure, plant-based foods, I'm connected to the earth. To life. To the sun. To the stars and moon. To animals. I feel precious interconnections that are impossible to take for granted. I'm experiencing—and deeply connected to—a planet that is alive. It might sound hokey, but trust me—it's real! Just wait—you'll see for yourself.

I have to laugh when people doubt or make negative assumptions about my lifestyle. Living this way is like having a secret key that opens the door to life at its best.

I think what really happens is that when overly skeptical, critical, or doubting people learn about raw food, they suddenly experience a deep fear that they might be making the "wrong" choices with respect to their own food and how they're feeding their families. Most people do not like to admit they're wrong, especially not about something as fundamental, primal, and emotional as food. It's like telling people they don't know how to tie their shoes or they don't know how to raise their kids properly. It's hard for people to acknowledge that their diet might be the reason they're not feeling well. Many people don't want to hear that. They're turned off by raw food before taking the chance to get turned on to it. I try to live as an example, hoping people will take notice and start asking questions. And, you know what? Many do!

Regardless of a person's age or what they have believed for years, there exists a fundamental truth: We are responsible for our own health, and we have a choice. We can use nutrition and food to help ourselves or hurt ourselves. Will you use your diet to weaken your body or strengthen it? Will your food and lifestyle choices accelerate your aging or slow it down? Hasten your death or prolong your life?

If you are not feeling well and you think that every day you should feel energetic and amazing, then perhaps it is time to try something new. Go for it—add more raw food to your life and see what happens. Harness the power of produce!

THE MEANING OF HEALTH

If you want to know the meaning and value of health, just ask someone who does not have it. Take a walk around a hospital. There is nothing like seeing fear in the eyes of someone who is ill, and in the eyes of those they love, to quickly snap you out of the delusion that health is to be taken for granted.

YOUR HEALTH: OWN IT!

Your health is your responsibility and no one else's. This is important. Your health is not your family's responsibility, or your doctor's, or the government's, and it's not a higher being's responsibility. It is yours. The sooner you recognize it and accept this, the better your life will be. Your daily choices matter. Become empowered and take control of your health.

It was a revelation when I discovered this simple fact: I can control what I eat. I can't control some other aspects of my life, such as traffic, weather, or other people, but I can control what I eat. Interestingly, eating a healthful diet makes dealing with those other stresses in life easier. I have seen people turn their lives around by changing how and what they eat, and you can, too. As you become mindful of what you put into your body, you immediately improve your life. The best part is that it's not something you have to wait for. You can start to feel the benefits within hours. When you start eating raw, you'll immediately notice that you no longer have to "recover" after eating, as you used to when you ate heavy, bloating foods. It is time to stop insulting your body, because you are all you have.

And you're not the only beneficiary. Always keep in mind that when someone becomes ill, it affects more than just that person. It affects the person's family and the people around him or her.

THE FOOD HEALTH LADDER

To think about society's food choices, picture a ladder going from least healthy at the bottom to healthiest at the top. At the very bottom of the ladder is what most Americans eat every day:

The S.A.D.

At the very bottom of the food ladder, you'll find the people who eat what is widely referred to as the "Standard American Diet"—appropriately referred to as S.A.D., because it is truly sad.

The S.A.D. comprises animal and plant products, in particular, foods containing nutritionally deficient processed ingredients that are high in sugars/starches, fats, cholesterol, chemicals, and preservatives. Imagine shoveling down sweetened cereals for breakfast, fast food for lunch, and hot dogs or pork chops for dinner, and you've got the picture. Those who eat this way may know they're eating badly, but their personal priorities do not place value on short- or long-term health.

The F.*.C.K.E.D. Diet

One step up from the S.A.D. diet is one that I've not so tongue-in-cheekly named the "Food Understanding Corrupted, Killing Even Doctors" diet.

This is the diet eaten by most Americans who think they are eating healthfully: chicken instead of beef, grilled instead of fried, skim milk instead of 2 percent, whole-grain bread instead of white bread. Does this sound like anyone you know? It should; it describes the vast majority of people who try at all to "eat healthy" in our society. It's how your doctor tells you to eat, as though anything healthier is just too impractical to prescribe. Unfortunately, people on this diet have a false sense of security, because diets rich in animal-based proteins and fats have been linked to higher mortality rates.

In a way, this is the saddest diet of all, because most of these people really, truly, are trying to eat well, but they are lacking something fundamental: information about what is healthful and what is not. Here is the problem: They receive information from the media and their doctors in terms of *relative* health—relative to the horribly disease-ridden S.A.D. baseline—not about what is truly optimal for the human body based on all available data.

Most health studies conducted in the United States assume that Americans will never change their habits dramatically, so they don't even bother to look into things that sound extreme to the uninformed majority. Such is the case with Harvard's famous long-range Nurses' Health Study, linking diet with diseases like breast cancer over the lifetime of those studied. With more than 350,000 participants, it is one of the largest studies of its kind, but it neglects to look at cases in which women consume only plant-based foods, based on the flawed circular reasoning that most people will never eat that way because they don't today. The false implication is that a relatively high incidence of many diseases is simply unavoidable. This is good science at its worst!

For a full account of this problem, I highly recommend T. Colin Campbell's life-changing book *The China Study*, which makes a brilliant case causally linking Western (animal-based) diets with Western diseases. This may not be news to you if you're reading this book, but what will make you angry is the media's reluctance to report Campbell's rigorous peer-reviewed findings. Most doctors don't even know about it. Here is a quote from Campbell's book:

> Professor Walter Willett (chair of Harvard University's Department of Nutrition) and I have had discussions about the findings [of the Nurses' Health Study] . . . I have always made the same point: whole foods, plant-based diets . . . are not included in the Nurses' Health Study cohort, and these types of diets are most beneficial to our health. Professor Willett has said to me, in response, on more than one occasion, "You may be right, Colin, but people don't want to go there."

Dr. Campbell continues: "Scientists should not be ignoring ideas just because we perceive that the public does not want to hear them. Consumers have the ultimate choice of whether to integrate our findings into their lifestyles, but we [scientists] owe it to them to give them the best information possible with which to make that decision and not decide for them."

So while the typical gym-going Americans ordering the "heart-smart" item on the menu think they are taking adequate control of their health, the truth is, the vast majority of their diets get a Grade D when compared to the range of dietary choices that are available, as opposed to those imposed upon us by an entrenched system of habits, social norms, agricultural subsidies, biased policy-makers, and self-perpetuating ignorance.

The Vegetarian Diet

Next on the ladder, a notch healthier, are vegetarians. Just so there's no confusion, vegetarians don't eat animal flesh (red meat, chicken, fish, etc.), but they do eat animal by-products, most notably eggs, milk, cheese, and other dairy products.

Because milk, cheese, and eggs contain many of the same harmful things, such as cholesterol and often hormones, that make meat unhealthful to eat, this cannot be considered a particularly healthy diet. In fact, I usually advise people who want to change gradually to cut out dairy and egg yolks even before meat!

The Vegan Diet

A step up on the ladder from vegetarians are vegans. Unlike vegetarians, vegans, by definition, don't consume any animal products or by-products (including honey in many cases). In fact, strictly speaking, true vegans don't wear or use animal products either, such as leather or wool or even pearls, based on a philosophical belief about animals' well-being. That said, in everyday vernacular, the word *vegan* often refers only to one's diet. As more people switch to a plant-based diet primarily for health reasons (and, increasingly, ecological awareness), it is more and more common to find self-described vegans who still consume honey, wear leather, etc.

It would be technically more accurate if they said they eat "a plant-based diet."

Is the distinction between vegetarian and vegan just splitting hairs? Definitely not; the leap from vegetarian to vegan is more profound than the leap from omnivore to vegetarian. Because eggs and dairy are chemically similar to meat, a vegetarian diet is not very different from a meat-eating diet from a health perspective.

From a lifestyle perspective, veganism requires a bigger adjustment than vegetarianism because it's easy to order something without meat in most restaurants, whereas milk, eggs, cheese, butter, cream, and so on are added to more dishes than you might have ever realized. Many servers, chefs, and restaurateurs do not understand what a vegan diet is, let alone offering options for vegans on the menu. One of the biggest adaptations vegans must make is learning where to eat and how to order from a non-vegan-friendly menu. Fortunately, this is a learnable skill and, with some practice, it becomes second nature.

And the results are worth it. Vegans who get a lot of fruits and vegetables in their diets (as opposed to "junk food vegans," who drink Cokes and eat Oreos, fries, and other highly processed foods) live long, healthy, vibrant lives. Going vegan is really the lowest rung you want to be on the ladder if you are truly serious about taking control of your health and grading yourself against what is possible, rather than against a baseline that accepts disease as unavoidable and something to be treated after the fact with drugs.

Here are some startling statistics from John Robbins' best-selling book *The Food Revolution*:

- Average cholesterol level in the United States: 210
- Average cholesterol level of U.S. vegetarians: 161
- Average cholesterol level of U.S. vegans: 133
- Average weight of vegan adults compared to non-vegetarian adults: 10 to 20 pounds (4.5 to 9 kg) lighter

THE HIGH-RAW DIET VS. THE ALL-RAW DIET

Just a few years ago, many people would have said that veganism was at the top of the healthy-eating ladder. But now we realize there is still something better: raw food.

At the top of the ladder of food health are people who eat either a "high-raw" diet or an "all-raw" diet. These terms refer to food that is 100 percent plant-based/vegan, often organic, and never heated above 118°F (48°C). "All raw" is what it sounds like: 100 percent raw. Because eating all raw is very difficult for most people to maintain indefinitely, raw fooders have invented the term "high raw" to signify a more common and feasible diet of about 70 to 85 percent raw food.

The leap from vegan to high raw or all raw is substantial, both in terms of health benefits and lifestyle impact, but it is made easier by two important things. First, high raw's health impacts can be felt immediately. We're not talking about avoiding heart disease down the road (you may have already done that by going vegan); we're talking about more energy, more vitality, restful sleep, clear skin, good digestion, and so on—right away! It's very exciting. (Actually, in addition to the short-term benefits, raw food's high concentration of phytonutrients and antioxidants is an excellent defense against cancer, and may be the single best reason for making the leap.)

Second, unlike going vegan, which is often done all the way or not at all, going raw can be more gradual. You can start eating 10 percent of your meals as raw, and gradually work your way up to 25 percent, 50 percent, and so on. In fact, it is this gradient aspect that necessitated the need for the term "high raw." (Most of the raw fooders I know are high raw, including myself.)

Which is healthier, high raw or all raw? There are scientific arguments for each, and more research is being done all the time. Personally, I have experienced great health by eating both ways. I think it depends on the individual, and that you should try each for yourself to see which style of raw you prefer. Perhaps you'll like to do both, alternating periodically or at different times of the year (cooked food helps keep you warm during colder months). Some people like to start out with an all raw-diet to jump-start their new healthy lifestyle, or to reach a weight-loss goal, and later ease into a high-raw diet that is more sustainable for the long run. (It is easier to get calories in cooked foods, largely because grain-based starchy foods are available if you're high raw, but not if you're all raw—you'd never eat raw flour, for instance. For this reason, it's easier to lose weight if you're all raw.)

The fact that some nutrients are released through cooking certain foods would support an argument for a high-raw diet over a strict all-raw diet in the long run. But keep in mind that while cooking makes some nutrients available to you, it also destroys others in the heating process.

Baby Steps

Every little change you make for the better will help get you to the next higher step on the ladder, and that means improvement. There is no need to jump from the bottom to the top all at once. In fact, it's often difficult for people to do that. The point of this book is to support you on every step, be it a baby step or a big leap, as you move into greater health in your life. If you're at the bottom and you remove, say, dairy from your diet, that's a huge step. You move higher on the ladder of health. Congratulations! Then, you remove meat and you move even higher, as you continue to experience greater health. Or, maybe you're a vegan and you eat a lot of flour-based, starchy foods. A step up the ladder would be to eat more fresh vegetables and fruits. Or, maybe your diet is 50 percent raw and you want to reach 75 percent raw.

The point is that you don't want to focus on the high ladder in front of you—just concentrate on the next step. That one step is the only thing that matters right now.

One Size Does Not Fit All with Raw

You don't need to go 100 percent raw to feel some great benefits. As I mentioned earlier, I usually eat a high-raw diet, which means I might eat mostly raw during the day but have a dinner that is part raw and part cooked. Or, perhaps I'm traveling and eat more cooked foods out of convenience (although raw on the road is definitely possible). There are times during the year, usually in January, where I will go 100 percent raw for a month or so, and then start easing back into high-raw territory again. Once the warm summer months hit, though, I'm usually back to 100 percent raw for a while. As the cooler weather comes back, I enjoy some cooked foods. All of this is to say that I have extended periods where I'm all raw and times when I'm not. Sometimes I have decaf organic coffee even though my day is filled with all raw foods. Sometimes I alternate a week of eating all raw with a week of high raw, and back again, week by week. It just depends, and that's the point. I'm flexible with it and I think I've found a perfect balance that way.

I have learned through the years that my body doesn't want cooked foods for very long, even if the food is considered healthful, like whole grains and steamed veggies. My body always directs me back to raw. This is a common experience among raw fooders; once they've adjusted to the lifestyle, it seems to become their new long-term baseline lifestyle. Even if they drift from time to time, the purity of raw food and the memory of how good it feels to eat it exerts a constant gravity that inevitably pulls them back.

Going raw doesn't have to be intimidating or hard. It's not about being a die-hard purist (perfection can be difficult for even the best-intentioned). It's about your purpose and progress—heading in a direction that is better for you, your family, animals, and the earth.

Take the first step in faith. You don't have to see the whole staircase, just take the first step.
—Martin Luther King Jr.

Now That I'm Going Raw, What Are All These Different Raw Diets I Hear About?

There are a lot of different opinions in the raw-food world. Don't be put off or confused by this, because it's part of the beauty of the raw vegan diet. There are many options, and one size does not have to fit all. *Ideal* changes from person to person and situation by situation. This is exciting because it allows variety to be a part of each person's diet.

Don't get caught up or stressed about certain ingredients or styles of eating raw. While you're learning more about raw food, you'll undoubtedly come across raw purists who eschew many things that sound interesting to you. Personally, I don't go down that road. For instance, some raw fooders will tell you to stay away from chocolate, even raw chocolate. Oh, hell no—I'd rather die! I say that if you enjoy raw chocolate, then keep enjoying it. If you like vinegar in your salad dressing, then use it. If you want coconut oil in your smoothies, then go for it. As with many things, you'll find people singing the praises of certain things and people who avoid them. You're not going to have any problems if you keep things balanced and eat a broad range of ingredients. If you question a particular ingredient, then do some research and decide for yourself if you want to increase it, decrease it, abstain from it, or make it your middle name.

The raw diet offers plenty of variety. During one season I can follow low-fat raw vegan principles by eating mostly fruits and greens, and in another season I can nourish my body with avocados, nuts, seeds, and divine raw vegan desserts. I love this flexibility and versatility. There are so many options. You can be a sproutarian for a spell. You can follow the fruitarian way of life at another time. You can explore green smoothies and juices and all things liquid—detox, anyone? You can nourish your body with loads of essential fatty acids and healthful fats from whole nuts, avocados, coconut, etc. You can pursue a natural-hygiene approach (much like a fruitarian) and avoid oils, garlic, and fermented foods.

Have fun with it and enjoy the variety that awaits your ride on the raw food train. Congratulate yourself for taking your health into your own hands and trying this healthy lifestyle, no matter which path you pursue on your journey with raw foods. Be confident that you're feeding your body wonderful nutrient-dense raw vegan foods, whether they're avocados, hemp seeds, pineapple, kale salads, gourmet raw foods, or a giant spoonful of Cheezy Hemp Nacho Sauce (those of you who regularly follow my blog know of my addiction to this—see the recipe on page 173). There are so many choices for you. There is no need to have to follow one plan.

The trick is simple: Listen to your body! Be patient and follow your intuition. Recognize that we are all different—we are different ages, starting from different points, from different backgrounds, living in different parts of the world, experiencing different environmental toxins, with different levels of stress and different levels of physical exercise.

Many people thrive on a 100 percent raw diet while keeping it balanced by rotating their greens and fruits, eating seasonally when possible, and supplementing as needed for any nutritional deficiencies they might have. (One way to be sure all your nutritional bases are covered is to have your blood analyzed annually and check on your levels of B_{12}, iodine, iron, vitamin D, and so on.) Other people thrive on a high-raw diet because it is less stressful to not have to eat raw at every meal.

We can all benefit by adding more raw, organic, vegan, high-nutrient whole foods to our lives, no matter where we currently are on the food-health ladder. I urge you to experiment and find the level of eating raw that works for you.

Nothing is worth more than this day.
—Goethe

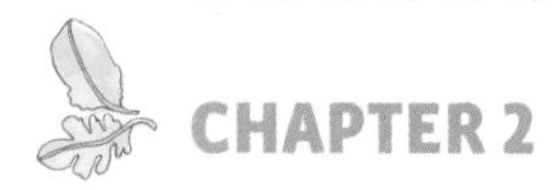

CHAPTER 2

THE HEALTH LANDSCAPE TODAY

The main health challenges for Americans today are diabetes, heart disease, cancer, obesity, osteoporosis, and depression. You won't find these same challenges in all parts of the world, but you will find them wherever people eat the typical Western diet. Tragically, these diseases are appearing in large numbers for the first time ever in cultures that are adopting the Western diet of animal-based foods.

If you look at cultures with the highest longevity, you will find that they do not even have words in their vocabulary for some of the diseases we are afflicted with here in the United States. Heart disease, cancer, diabetes, obesity, osteoporosis, and depression are practically unknown in those parts of the world. We might as well refer to our American eating habit as "The Suicide Diet," because this way of eating is the biggest cause of disability, disease, and death in the United States today.

Much of the food consumed in America will support life, but it won't support health. There is a difference between just enduring versus living life to the fullest and loving every day of it because you are truly healthy. A lot of people don't realize the potential well-being they could experience because they've never felt that way before. It falls into the category of "you don't know what you don't know."

There have been many cases of people who have stopped, and even reversed, their poor health by eating a raw plant-based diet. Our bodies are amazing. In fact, that statement doesn't even do our bodies justice. Our bodies are freakin' phenomenal! Did you know that you are made up of over a hundred trillion cells? A hundred trillion! So, why not feed them the nutrients they need to thrive? When your cells become diseased, they behave in abnormal ways, many of which bring on much pain and suffering. Eating a diet that is high in raw food can help you fight disease and maintain a healthy immune system.

Henry Bieler, M.D., author of *Food Is Your Best Medicine*, said one of the first questions a woman asks after giving birth is, "Doctor, is my baby all right?" He was puzzled by this because he believed that if every mother's desire is to have a truly healthy baby, she would take better care of herself before getting pregnant and during her pregnancy.

AMERICA'S HEALTH CHALLENGES

Heart Disease

It is no secret that heart disease and cancer are two hallmarks of animal-based diets. As of 2007, heart disease was the leading cause of death in the United States. I'll bet this comes as no surprise—you can probably rattle off the names of people you know who've suffered from conditions related to heart disease.

But did you know that it's preventable and even reversible? It's frustrating, because people can actually do something about their heart disease, yet so many people don't. It's amazing how quickly people can recover from heart disease by diet alone.

Studies show that a single bad meal can cause injury to your arteries. Dr. Caldwell Esselstyn of the Cleveland Clinic, one of the world's leading authorities on reversing heart disease through diet, says that when it comes to cholesterol, "moderation kills." When asked about the effects of an occasional steak or slice of pizza, Dr. Esselstyn says, "We now know that a single fatty meal compromises coronary flow. This is true even in young people. You can see it with a scan five minutes later."

Our livers produce all the cholesterol we need, and one of the great things about plants is that they contain zero cholesterol. So many people think they are doing their bodies a favor by eating chicken instead of red meat (to reduce cholesterol), but it isn't so. Chicken has approximately the same amount of cholesterol as red meat. It is simple. Avoid meat.

The risk of developing heart disease among meat-eaters is 50 percent higher than among vegetarians. According to William Castelli, M.D., director of the Framingham Heart Study, the longest-running clinical study in medical history, vegans "have the lowest rates of coronary disease of any group in the country . . . they have a fraction of our heart attack rate, and they have only 40 percent of our cancer rate." He also states, "We've never had a heart attack in Framingham in thirty-five years in anyone who had a cholesterol level under 150."

And . . . one last note . . . let's talk about sex, baby! If the Standard American Diet (high in saturated fat and cholesterol) can block arteries to the heart, brain, and all other parts of the body, it should not be surprising that the same diet can block arteries to the entire genital region. Yes, erectile dysfunction (ED) is commonly caused by lack of blood flow and blocked arteries, typically the result of consuming meat and animal by-products (eggs and dairy).

According to a study by the U.S. National Institute on Aging, cholesterol levels are a bigger factor than age in the onset of impotence. And according to the Joslin Diabetes Center at Harvard University, "Diabetes can cause nerve and artery damage in the genital area, disrupting the blood flow necessary for an erection."

Don't let meat destroy your health or ruin your love life. It's not worth it!

Diabetes

Diabetes is a condition where the body cannot efficiently metabolize certain foods, most notably starches and sugars, as a result of a dirty circulatory system.

A March 2003 study published in the journal *Diabetes Care* estimated the costs of diabetes in the United States in 2002 at $132 billion, with direct medical costs totaling $92 billion. That's a lot of money. And of all the drug-dosage errors made in hospitals in this country, the greatest number of errors is made with insulin, because it's tricky trying to figure out the right amount to administer.

The good news is that the potential we have for preventing diabetes is astounding. A whopping 90 to 95 percent of all cases of type-2 diabetes are preventable and even reversible! Check out Rawfor30days.com to see a mind-blowing documentary about a group of diabetic patients helping to heal their diabetic conditions with a raw plant-based diet. It is exhilarating and inspiring.

Cancer

Cancer is scary. I have seen close family and friends suffer with this terrible disease, much of it needlessly. In the United States, breast cancer is at an alarmingly high rate. More and more evidence shows that eating animal protein increases your risk of getting this terrible disease. According to Karen Emmons, M.D., of the Dana-Farber Cancer Institute in Boston, "5 to 10 percent of all cancers are caused by inherited genetic mutations. By contrast, 70 to 80 percent have been linked to [diet and other] behavioral factors."

What we know is this: Cancer thrives in an acidic environment where there is a lack of oxygen. When you eat food that is acidic by nature, such as animal protein, you make your bloodstream more acidic. Hence, to help prevent cancer, or fight it if you already have it, limit foods that raise your acidity level, and increase alkaline foods (fresh raw plant foods).

Obesity

A team at Johns Hopkins University in Baltimore examined twenty studies, and Dr. Youfa Wang, who led the study, said in a statement, "Obesity is a public health crisis. If the rate of obesity and overweight continues at this pace, by 2015, 75 percent of adults and nearly 24 percent of U.S. children and adolescents will be overweight or obese."

Peter Steinberg, M.D., a well-known radiologist in Arizona, gave the following speech in 2007 at a continuing-medical-education seminar where the focus was wellness, diet, and lifestyle.

> A topic on everyone's mind today is how to achieve health, or in some cases, how to maintain it. On a daily basis, newspapers and magazines are filled with articles on health, diet, and nutrition. Vitamins, diet supplements, and potions of all sorts are espoused as elixirs for a long, healthy life. With this tidal wave of information, it's often difficult to separate truth from fiction.
>
> Compounding all of this information and misinformation is the problem of obesity in this country. Sixty-five percent of the U.S. adult population (twenty years and older) is either overweight or obese. More frightening, 16 percent of children and teens in this country, according to the American Heart Association, are overweight. It is a problem that is not going away. In fact, it is accelerating. In 1993, not a single state in the union reported an obesity prevalence rate above 20 percent. Ten years later in 2003, thirty-one states had obesity prevalence rates between 20 and 24 percent and another four states had rates at or above 25 percent.
>
> Clearly, we are in the middle of an obesity epidemic and this will result in more cardiovascular disease (already the number-one killer), diabetes, hypertension, cancer, degenerative joint disease, etc. Some suggest that if we continue along this same path, the current generation of children could be the first in American history to live shorter lives than their parents.
>
> There are financial consequences to obesity—costs that we all share as individuals, employers and through government-sponsored health programs such as Medicaid and Medicare.

Medical expenditures that result from treating obesity-related diseases are significant. According to R. Sturm et al., obese adults between the ages of 20 and 65 have annual medical expenses that are 36 percent higher than those of normal-weight people. As BMI (body mass index) increases so do the number of sick days, medical claims, and health-care costs. According to Thompson et al., the health-related economic cost to U.S. business is significant, representing about 5 percent of total medical care costs.

Allergies, Arthritis, Osteoporosis, and Dairy

I can't write a book about health and not include information about dairy. Dairy is linked with arthritis, heartburn, headaches, osteoporosis, obesity, heart disease, cancer, diabetes, acne, and more. It's often filled with hormones, steroids, antibiotics, and pesticides. It can even contain white blood cells from the cow—in other words, pus. And people drink it! That's quite the cocktail, to which I say, "No, thanks!"

Humans are designed to digest a mother's breast milk—as babies. We're the only species that consumes milk as adults. Hmmmm—think about it. Do you ever see anywhere in nature an animal that is past its youngest phase in life and is still attached to its mother's nipple? No. So why in the world do we continue to consume dairy when it's made for babies?

Dairy products are full of saturated fats and cholesterol. Often a body will develop a cold or "allergies" to fight the dairy invasion, which is why dairy forms mucus. All you have to do to test this is to give up all dairy for one week. That's it, just one week. Then, go eat a slice of pizza and have some ice cream and see what happens to you the next morning. You'll be filled with phlegm, snot, and mucus. Yuck. One of the reasons people have bad breath in the morning is from mucus coating their nasal passages and throat. The mucus is a result of undigested lactose and the acidic nature of pasteurized milk. Both of these encourage the growth of bacteria. According to the periodical *Pediatrics*, "Dairy products may play a major role in the development of allergies, asthma, sleep difficulties, and migraine headaches." I know many people who experienced immediate improvement with their allergies and asthma once they stopped consuming dairy. If you suffer from these ailments, try eliminating dairy and see how clearly you can breathe, starting within just a couple of days!

And don't forget about all of the drugs added to cows' milk that isn't certified as organic. According to the Physicians Committee for Responsible Medicine's *Good Medicine* magazine (Spring-Summer 2011), "In 2009, 29 million pounds of antibiotics were used to raise animals in factory farms, according to a recent Food and Drug Administration report. Animal agriculture accounts for about 80 percent of the antibiotic use in the United States and is increasingly blamed for the growing resistance to antibiotics among disease-causing bacteria." Yuck!

Arthritis is another problem for many Americans, and as baby boomers enter their older years, this problem will only get worse. Dairy can aggravate arthritis terribly. In controlled studies, dairy products are the most frequently cited food triggers of arthritis. (Has the Dairy Council—which spends millions of dollars on advertising to convince us that we need their product—ever made any TV ads telling you that their product actually triggers allergies and arthritis?)

My mom used to suffer from arthritis pain on a daily basis until she eliminated dairy from her diet. There was a time when she couldn't stand up without experiencing arthritic pain. Once she stopped consuming dairy, she started to feel improvement within a matter of days.

For people who are concerned about getting enough calcium to prevent osteoporosis and are using milk as a means to that end, read this: There is not one study that has found dairy consumption to be a deterrent to osteoporosis. On the contrary, many doctors and experts in the field have shown that the high-protein content of dairy actually leaches calcium from the body.

Because protein is acidic to the body, in order to help alkalize the bloodstream, calcium is taken from the bones and added to the blood. It is no surprise that the countries showing the highest consumption of dairy and meat also have the highest incidence of osteoporosis and hip fractures.

Eskimos, who eat a lot of protein, have some of the highest rates of osteoporosis in the world. According to Neal Barnard, the president of the Physicians Committee for Responsible Medicine, "Animal protein is one of the biggest predictors of kidney failure and osteoporosis," and that includes dairy.

You don't need animal foods to get your calcium needs met if you're eating a healthy raw, plant-based diet. When you gobble up a diet full of fresh veggies, fruits, nuts, and seeds, you will satisfy your calcium requirements. Again, it bears repeating that equally as important, by eliminating or drastically reducing your animal product consumption you will make your bones and body stronger—because you won't be losing as much calcium in your urine. Oh, and try this on for size: We absorb calcium more efficiently from vegetables. Hurray!

So what are some great sources of plant-based calcium? Kale, collard greens, mustard greens, cabbage, kelp, seaweed, watercress, broccoli, fruits, nuts, and seeds. You also obtain much higher levels of manganese, chromium, magnesium, and selenium from fresh fruits and vegetables. It really is that simple. If you need a substitute for dairy

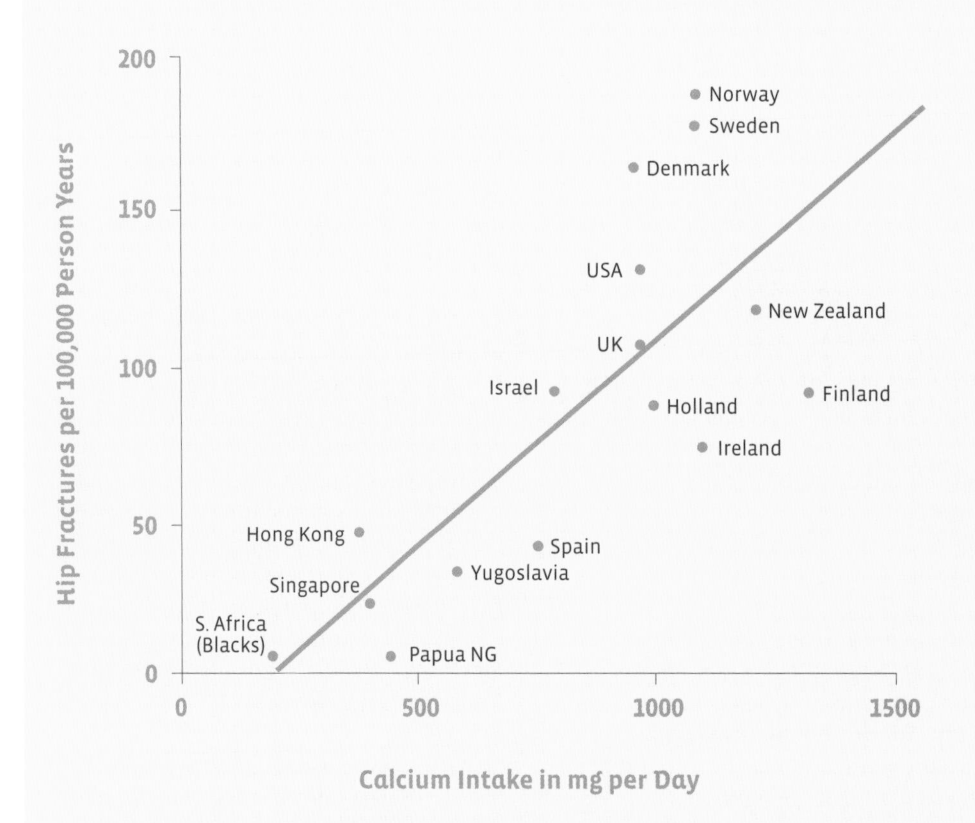

"Populations that consume the most cow's milk and other dairy products have among the highest rates of osteoporosis and hip fracture."

Source: Abelow, Holford and Insogna (1992)

when eating cereal or raw granola, then try raw nut or seed milk (Raw Almond Milk is my favorite; see recipe on page 177). This is the most delicious and healthy substitute for unhealthful cow's milk any day. To learn more, check out MilkSucks.com.

Stress

Stress creates an acidic condition in the body, which can be a breeding ground for disease. There will always be stress in our lives to some degree, but we can help minimize the effect it has on us physically by eating a diet that is high in raw foods. Specifically, the nutrients that help us combat stress are vitamin C, B-complex vitamins, calcium, magnesium, and digestive enzymes. Eating a varied and well-balanced raw plant-based diet helps ensure you get plenty of these vitamins and minerals.

Depression

Depression is a horrible mental state that afflicts numerous Americans today. As a result, prescriptions for treating this disease are at an all-time high. I am a firm believer that the chemicals found in a lot of processed foods today do wacky things to our brain chemistry and can easily contribute to depression. According to *Good Medicine* magazine (Spring–Summer 2011), "Consumption of foods containing saturated fats and trans fats may contribute to depression, according to new research. Scientists in Spain analyzed the diets of more than 12,000 people for six years and found that those who ate the most trans fats had a 48 percent higher risk of depression, compared to those who did not eat trans fats."

That is why so many people immediately notice an improvement in their mood once they start eliminating junk from their diets and start eating fresh, vibrant plant foods. It's no secret that people report a marked increase in happiness, mental clarity, and focus when they go raw.

But there is a less well-known, and perhaps more important, psychological benefit to going raw. It's an effect that is harder to grasp and fully comprehend until it happens to you personally. If you are new to raw food, the following may sound strange and a little "out there," but many people describe a new and hard-to-define sense of "connection" with their food once they go raw. And by extension, they feel a new and different connection to their world, nature, and the role we have on this planet. Imagine feeling truly connected! To everything! The effects of this take many forms. It's not at all uncommon, for instance, for people to want to start growing some of their own food. Even people living in high-rise apartments! To many, going raw is like awakening something deep within that has always been there, but has been suppressed.

Now, maybe this quasi-spiritual, transformational experience is the product of simply thinking more about what you put into your body. Or maybe it's a by-product of having a healthier, cleaner, toxin-free internal state, which makes you simply feel good. Or it's a result of sleeping well, maybe for the first time in years. But regardless, in many ways, the food we eat is by far (even more so than the air we breathe) the most direct connection we have to the outside world. The molecules we ingest actually become us. The old adage is true: "You are what you eat." Literally.

Antiaging: Physically and Mentally

Age prematurely? No, thank you. I want to slow down the aging process naturally as much as I can. It makes sense that raw foods can help. You'll see that most people who are living the raw lifestyle have a beautiful glow about them, with soft skin and typically far fewer wrinkles than other people the same age. I attribute this to all of the nutrition they're getting from eating antioxidant-rich foods, as well as by eliminating foods that are acidic and hard on the body (animal flesh, animal by-products, cholesterol, processed foods, high-sugar and high-fat foods). Start living the raw lifestyle and you just might find yourself spending a lot less money on fancy antiwrinkle creams, which are full of potentially hazardous chemicals anyway. It's like getting a face-lift by living the raw lifestyle—and you've gotta love that!

Where aging is concerned, another horrible challenge in our world today has to do with people suffering from Alzheimer's disease. The raw lifestyle can help here, too. A study in the *American Journal of Medicine* showed that people in their study who drank an 8-ounce (250-ml) glass of fruit or vegetable juice three or more times a week were 76 percent less likely to develop Alzheimer's than those who drank less than one serving. It's those powerful antioxidants and phytonutrients going to work for you all the time.

Sleep Problems

Aside from eating well and exercising, getting enough sleep is one of the most important things you can do for health and longevity. Aim to get at least seven hours per night, ideally more like eight to ten hours. Sufficient sleep improves your mood, memory, cognitive function, reduces stress and inflammation, decreases risks for heart disease and cancer, and may even help you lose weight. Besides, sleep is just plain great! Your goal should be to get enough restful sleep that you wake up "naturally"—that is, without any stimulus such as an alarm clock, sounds, or having to pee. Raw food can help you achieve this sleep-abundant nirvana!

As a result of eating so much raw food, I have the best sleep ever. I used to think it was normal to wake up in the middle of the night drenched in sweat, even though I went to bed feeling chilly. I would toss and turn throughout the night, blaming my mattress for the unruly sleep. I believed that it was impossible to wake up feeling refreshed. Furthermore, I never imagined a life without my alarm clock—that was crazy talk. Sleeping is when your body repairs the wear and tear that happens during the day. This means you must fill your body with the nutrients required to nurture and enable these repair processes. Eating right not only helps you sleep better, it makes sleep more productive in contributing to your ongoing health.

Do you want to wake up refreshed (with or without an alarm clock), ready to bounce out of bed and start the day—without needing caffeine? Restful sleep helps you do this, and in order for your body to get the best sleep, you can't fill it with toxic sludge. End of story.

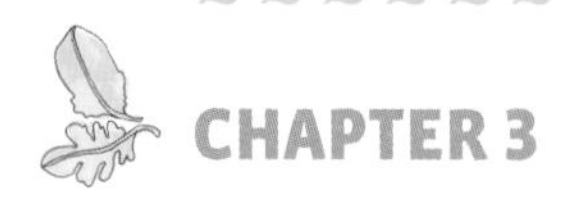

CHAPTER 3

HOW RAW WORKS

After reading the following information about enzymes, nutrients, and the detrimental effect heat can have on your food, you will realize what a no-brainer it is that raw food should be the majority of your diet. It just makes sense.

Raw food is healthful for two reasons: (1) It contains phytonutrients (nutrients found in plants); (2) it promotes digestion due to its fiber, water, and enzyme content.

Phytonutrients and enzymes are damaged by high levels of heat; enzymes start to "denature" (become mangled) around 118°F (48°C)[1]. At higher temperatures, phytonutrients start to become less bio-available, depending on the temperature, duration, cooking method, and other factors[2].

PHYTONUTRIENTS

The most fundamental component of the raw food lifestyle and the reason it is so healthy is that it contains vitamins and phytonutrients. These plant nutrients (also known as phytochemicals), are biologically active compounds that help the body to fight and prevent disease. These smart little helpers are starting to get much more recognition today among scientists and, to some extent, the media (and one day, maybe, policy-makers). They are known to fight directly against viruses and bacteria, as well as promote a healthy immune system and help to fight the process of aging. No wonder all those raw-food vegans look so young and vibrant!

Scientists are constantly discovering more and more important facts about phytonutrients. Did you know that there are substances in broccoli sprouts that sweep toxins out of cells? And that the material in nuts can help prevent damage to cells' DNA? Plus, certain phytonutrients can inhibit the activation of specific cancer genes. I mean, *wow!* Give me some phytonutrient-packed raw-food goodness!

The effects of phytonutrients are far-reaching and also play a critical role for children with respect to their future, beginning in the womb when the mother is pregnant, according to many nutrition experts.

I'm so glad that I ate phyto-nutrient-packed foods while I was pregnant and breastfeeding, and that I continue to feed those foods to my family. I'm setting up my family for a life of good health. What a gift!

In case you're not convinced yet, although I suspect you are with all of this amazing information, phytonutrients are where the party is. Beta-carotene (think apricots and carrots) helps give your skin a glow, and carotenoids (in orange and yellow produce) can reduce your risk for breast cancer. The silica in cucumbers (one of my favorites!) is great for connective tissue and collagen. Lycopene (think not only tomatoes, but also watermelon, pink grapefruit, and papaya) helps to prevent and treat various cancers, heart disease, cataracts, and more. Doesn't all of this amazing information make you want to run to the refrigerator and gorge on some fresh raw produce?

I could go on and on about how amazing phytonutrients are and how important they are for protecting your body against diseases and illness. Every time I read one of these studies or see something online about the powers of such-and-such a phytonutrient I'm grateful for my decision to live this lifestyle because I'm getting all of them, and much more, without having to obsess endlessly about whether I'm getting enough. By eating a diet primarily comprising raw plant-based foods, believe me, I get plenty!

One of the most important functions of phytonutrients is their antioxidant capacity. Antioxidants help fight free radicals in the body, which damage the cells and accelerate aging. A study from UCLA/Louisiana State University of more than 17,500 men and women showed that the consumption of raw vegetables correlates with higher levels of folic acid, vitamins C and E, lycopene, and alpha and beta-carotene in the bloodstream. Another study, from the *American Journal of Clinical Nutrition*, shows that apples and pears help to fight heart disease due to their high levels of flavonoids, which are anti-inflammatory and support a healthy heart.

The problem with phytonutrients, however, is that most are heat sensitive and become less available to the body when cooked. So, if you eat cooked veggies and think you are getting lots of phytonutrients and vitamins, think again. Many of these valuable elements have been destroyed.

One of the ways fresh organic raw food helps you get to and maintain your perfect weight is that it is full of nutrients, which most people are typically starved of. When eating a diet of mostly cooked food, people often find themselves hungry, because their bodies need not more calories, but more nutrients.

Last but not least, phytonutrients are responsible for giving fruits and vegetables their gorgeous, vibrant colors. This makes them pleasing to the eye, which is important for your mind-set. In real estate, they say it's all about "location, location, location"—well, when it comes to food, it's all about "presentation, presentation, presentation." Raw plant-based breakfasts, lunches, and dinners, with all of their beautiful, radiant colors, please the eye as well as the appetite.

ENZYMES

Enzymes are the power of life; literally, the working machinery of every cell in our body. They are living forces that conduct and direct every activity within our cells. Enzymes are made of amino acids and are critical for life. Basically, without enzymes, you would cease to exist. However, heat deforms enzymes so they no longer function properly. Heat's effect on enzymes is analogous to bending a metal part of a machine, such as a car's engine. Once the part is bent, it can no longer do its job and the engine will break down.

It's often said that a person's digestive system indicates his or her level of health. Many raw fooders believe that cooked or processed foods, which are devoid of their natural enzymes, as well as water (lost in the heating process), are more difficult to digest. The idea is that the living (metabolically active) enzymes already present in plant-based foods help the body to digest, or break down foods, so that digestion is less taxing on your body's resources. An enzyme-rich diet is also thought to increase vitality and slow the aging process. That said, many nutritionists and doctors do not believe that enzymes present in food are necessary, as the body makes its own digestive enzymes to do the job. The truth remains however that we have barely begun to understand the role of even the thousands of enzymes our own bodies produce, let alone those from other sources. Suffice it to say that more research is needed to fully understand the role that enzymes already present in living food may have on digestion. One thing is for sure: my digestion is in top shape when I eat raw food and I have much more energy.

PROTEIN

For too long, we have been misguided and programmed to believe that the only source of protein is meat and dairy. In reality, plant-based foods contain plenty of high-quality protein that is easier for your body to digest. The reason they are higher quality is simple: Plant proteins are found inside plant cells, the walls of which are made of the rigid material we call fiber. Fiber passes through the system in a nice, orderly fashion, giving us healthy, regular bowel movements. In contrast, animal proteins are inside animal cells, the walls of which are made of cholesterol, and our bodies aren't well equipped to break these down. When absorbed into our blood, cholesterol makes our blood thick and clogs our arteries. In fact, cholesterol kills more Americans every year than anything else. By eating a wide variety of plants, including plenty of greens, it is very easy to get 100 percent "complete" protein, meaning that all eight essential amino acids are present in abundance. It's all about quality versus quantity when it comes to protein, because a high-protein diet can be dangerous.

Think of this: Even as a baby, when you are most in need of protein for rapid growth, your ideal food, human breast milk, which has been designed and optimized by millions of years of evolution, contains only about 2 percent protein. That is all babies need, and they have the highest need for protein of all humans, because they grow faster than at any other age. Coincidentally—or perhaps not so coincidentally—this percentage of protein is typically the same found in—guess what?—most fruits and vegetables.

Excess protein (in the form of animal products or by-products) can harm your digestive tract, steal calcium from your bones, drain you of energy, and cause you to gain weight. Moreover, high protein and fat consumption is linked to cancer, heart disease, arthritis, kidney and liver problems, osteoporosis, diabetes, and obesity.

How much protein does a person need? The World Health Organization (WHO) recommends that only about 10 percent of our calories come from protein (perhaps more if you are an athlete, pregnant, or breastfeeding). People are so concerned about getting enough protein that you'd think that protein deficiency was an actual problem in our culture. Huh? Where is this problem exactly? Show me somebody who doesn't get enough protein but otherwise eats enough food. Put it this way: In your whole life, have you ever met anybody (who isn't starving in general) who is protein deficient?

Protein deficiency is simply not part of our culture's reality. The world's longest-lived cultures, such as Okinawans and the Hunzas of Pakistan, who frequently live to be over one hundred years old, consume only small amounts of protein.

People often ask me about eating raw meat. While it is true that the enzymes are intact in raw meat, it introduces a host of other problems, most notably parasites and other poisons. Fish is especially dangerous. Heavy metals that pollute our oceans are absorbed by fish, making them toxic. The flesh of fish can accumulate toxins up to 9 million times as concentrated as those in the waters they live in. Additionally, farmed fish are often fed antibiotics. According to the Centers for Disease Control and Prevention, 325,000 people get sick and some die every year in the United States from eating contaminated seafood.

Carbohydrates should be loved, not feared. Glucose, the natural sugar found in plant foods, is the natural fuel for our bodies. Natural-sugar foods, such as fresh raw fruit, fuel our brain and most other bodily functions. Carbohydrates are therefore extremely important for the body. The best and most nutritious carbohydrates you can get are in the form of fruit and vegetables. (Note: Because they have seeds, cucumbers, tomatoes, zucchini, and other seed-bearing "vegetables" are considered non-sweet fruits rather than vegetables.)

Our cultural fear of carbohydrates exists because we have come to associate the word *carbohydrates* with what are sometimes called "empty carbs": nutritionally bankrupt foods such as white bread, pasta, cookies, cake, doughnuts, and so on. These foods are:

* Low in nutrition
* Low in fiber
* Low in water content
* Very high in calories
* Yummy to babies, who then become addicted for life, prompting us to invent the term *comfort food*

When you eat empty carbs, you are filling up not on good, necessary things like water and fiber but on almost pure starchy sugar. No wonder, then, that if you eat any of these foods until you "feel full," you will have eaten far more calories than you need to maintain your weight but still be deficient in essential nutrients, which leads you to quickly feel hungry again. Other than gulping down a few sticks of butter, eating these foods is perhaps the fastest way to create a caloric surplus, which is to say, gain fatty weight. (Your body converts and stores unused carbohydrates in the fat that deposits around your waist, butt—and heart.)

The important point is this: The carbohydrates found in fruits and vegetables are not to be feared. They come prepackaged in good proportions with other things that fill you up, signaling you to stop eating—specifically, fiber, water, and nutrients. Fiber and water take up a lot of room and physically make your stomach feel full. Stomach fullness is one of several of the body's satiety cues (along with blood sugar levels and jaw fatigue from chewing), causing your brain to tell you to stop eating. Consider fiber your new BFF! In contrast to empty calories, nutrients operate on longer time frames, such as hours or days: if you have enough of a given nutrient, your body typically stops craving foods high in that nutrient.

If controlling your weight is a problem, remember this one thing, and it will change your life: the trick to being able to eat a comfortable amount—essentially "as much as you feel like eating"—is to eat foods that fill you up with fiber and water rather than pure sugar or fat. In other words, fruits and vegetables. It boils down to the simple math of calories per unit of volume, because your stomach has a finite amount of space.

In practice, if you're trying to lose weight and you have a craving for something hearty and comforting, like spaghetti, first eat your fill of salad or drink a green smoothie. Once your stomach is full, the bad food won't seem nearly as appetizing. You've probably heard the advice given to people trying to lose weight that drinking a glass of water can help curb your appetite. Eating fruits or vegetables is taking that basic idea one step further, as fiber- and water-rich foods, aside from providing nutrition and being more satisfying than a glass of water, will stay in your stomach longer and prolong the effect of filling you up.

FATS

Raw plant fats are helpful in transitioning you to the raw lifestyle. The healthiest plant fats come in the form of whole foods, such as avocados, nuts, seeds, olives, and coconuts. "Good fats" can bind with toxins, helping to eliminate them from your body, making these some of the most healing fats for the body. If you are looking for essential fatty acids, then look no further than hemp foods, flaxseeds, chia seeds, walnuts, and leafy greens such as lettuce, broccoli, spinach, and kale. There is no need to turn to animal sources for fatty acids.

Within reason, you will not get fat by eating plant fats. The rule is still everything in moderation, of course—you can't eat ten avocados a day and expect to lose weight—but frequently eating sensible portions of these foods is not an issue for most people with respect to weight.

The bad fats people often consume include trans fats, saturated animal fats, and refined polyunsaturated fats, such as those found in refined cooking oils. But even good natural fats (hemp and flax, for example) are sensitive to heat and quickly damaged by it. Furthermore, heated fats lose their antioxidant qualities and are classified as carcinogenic. Keep it raw, folks!

Greens

If you want to improve your health, energy level, and overall well-being, then one of the most powerful things you can do is to add more nutrient-dense greens to your diet. They're amazing and the effect is fast.

Raw food devotees refer to greens as "nutritious excellence" because of their abundance of chlorophyll, phytonutrients, vitamins, and minerals. Chlorophyll is the green pigment molecule in plants responsible for absorbing the sun's energy for photosynthesis. The chlorophyll molecule in plants is chemically similar to hemoglobin in human blood. The only difference in the two molecules is that the central atom in chlorophyll is magnesium, whereas in humans it is iron. (Isn't that cool? We animals are more closely related to plants than you'd have thought.) As a food supplement, chlorophyll can detoxify and purify the blood and liver, help build red blood cells, and aid in tissue repair.

One of the most powerful green foods available is wheatgrass. This grass can be juiced and drunk straight (warning: it is intense!) or added to juice and smoothies. Wheatgrass that is certified organic produces very high concentrations of chlorophyll, enzymes, and vitamins. This plant has a nutrient profile similar to that of other leafy green vegetables and contains vitamins A, B complex, C, and E; the trace elements calcium, iron, magnesium, and potassium; enzymes; and amino acids. As an antioxidant, organic wheatgrass can boost the immune system and soak up free radicals. Organic wheatgrass has been shown to be a powerful body detoxifier. Its high chlorophyll content helps to cleanse the liver, tissues, and cells and purifies the blood. Organic wheatgrass also contains folic acid and iron, which are required for proper red blood cell production.

You'll find that chomping and chomping on endless amounts of greens results in masseter fatigue (a tired jaw muscle). Again, this is one of the body's satiety cues, meaning you'll naturally be inclined to stop eating. If you want more greens in your diet, but you are tired of chewing them, then two other options are (1) juice the greens, which extracts the fiber (plant pulp), allowing you to consume more greens, and therefore, more nutrients; or

(2) make green smoothies where you blend (in a blender) the greens, typically with some fruit to make them taste better.

I've been asked before whether it is possible to eat too many greens. In my opinion, balance is the key to everything. It is important to rotate the foods you eat, including greens. An easy way to do this is eating seasonal produce. Another way, for greens especially, is to vary the greens you eat each week.

1. Edward Howell. *Food Enzymes for Health and Longevity*. Lotus Press, 1994.

2. Emilia Leskova, et al. "Vitamin Losses: Retention During Heat Treatment and Continual Changes Expressed by Mathematical Models." *Journal of Food Composition and Analysis*. June 1, 2006.

CHAPTER 4

ORGANICS

Organic refers to the way agricultural products are grown and processed. The goal in organic farming is to grow healthy crops while maintaining and replenishing soil fertility without using toxic pesticides, herbicides, or fertilizers. *Certified organic* means the item has been grown in accordance with strict uniform standards that are verified by an independent state or private organization.

When you're shopping for organic produce, look for a five-digit code on it. If it starts with a zero, or is only four digits long, then it's not organic.

Dr. Alan Greene of Stanford's Children's Hospital neatly summarizes the argument for organics: "Eat organic produce. Your immune system won't waste energy trying to fight off the toxins that are sprayed on conventional fruits and vegetables."

Eating organics frees up your immune system to do its evolved job, which is to fight off pathogens, cancer, and other diseases originating from environmental sources. Your body's natural defense mechanisms are incredibly strong, but like anything else, they can only handle so much attack. To keep your defensive line from being spread too thin, you should therefore limit exposure to toxins (and stress) as much as possible. It's important to realize that consuming pesticides and herbicides—even if they have not been found to be directly carcinogenic—can, in effect, lead to cancer if they use up your supply of antioxidants, which would otherwise have prevented cancer that was generated by another source.

It's true that organic foods typically cost more than conventionally grown foods, but this may be true only in the short term. After you adopt a healthier lifestyle with healthier food choices, including organics, you may find yourself frequenting the doctor's office less and spending less on medications, both over-the-counter and prescription, not to mention that you may have a lower chance of dying prematurely.

Organically produced foods must meet rigorous governing regulations in all aspects of production. Organic food is labor- and management-intensive, and is usually produced on smaller farms, which don't benefit from economies of scale. These factors cause the cost to be higher. But as the saying goes, you get what you pay for. And remember that organic foods require more manual labor, such as removing pests by hand in some cases. This means that organic farmers are hit much harder than big factory farms by policies that restrict access to an adequate supply of migrant labor. Just something to keep in mind when you look at the price of food that hasn't been dowsed in carcinogenic chemicals.

We can all buy organic foods to prepare at home, but unfortunately, most restaurants don't use organic food—not yet, anyway. This is disappointing, but will change over time. If enough customers (read: you, your friends, your family, and so on) demanded organic every time they ordered food, more producers would produce it, and prices would come down. So, vote with your dollar! When you go to a restaurant and you're paying the bill, take a moment to fill out the comment card, or write directly on the receipt, that you would eat there more often if they offered some organic foods. Or, my favorite (and likely much more effective) trick, when your server takes your drink order, ask if they have any organic wines. If they do, consider ordering some (if you're of drinking age and not driving). If they don't, say, "Okay, I'll just have water." If this happened just three times a week, per waiter, per restaurant, then organic wines would be ubiquitous in restaurants in just a few months. Remember, you're the customer. Restaurant management can't read your mind. You must tell them what you want. This is how people can make a difference.

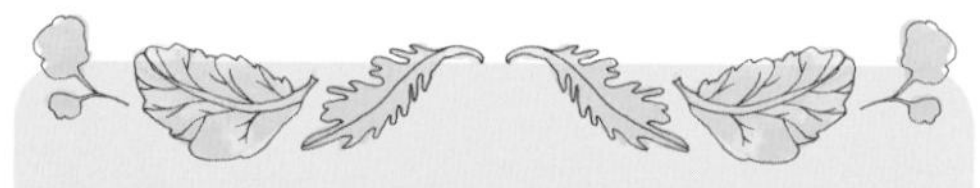

IS WINE VEGAN?

Many wines are not vegan. Animal-based products such as gelatin, egg whites, and casein are often used to remove impurities and clarify wine. Even though these additives are ultimately filtered out, the wine is not considered vegan. Look for "Vegan" on the label to be sure that no animal products were used in your wine's production.

TIPS FOR GOING ORGANIC ON A BUDGET

With a little extra planning, it is possible to eat organic without breaking the bank. Here are tips that will help you afford organic foods:

***Buy in bulk.** Ask the store you frequent if they'll give you a deal for buying foods by the case. (Just make sure it's a case of something you can go through in a timely fashion, so it doesn't get wasted.) Consider this for bananas (you can peel and freeze these) or greens, especially if you drink lots of smoothies or green juices.

***See if your neighbors, family, or friends will split the price of purchasing in bulk, such as buying certain foods by the case.** When you do this, you can go beyond your local grocery store and contact places like BoxedGreens.com or DiamondOrganic.com. Some sellers offer quantity discounts if your order goes over a certain amount or if you get certain foods by the case. Try this with anyone you buy from. It never hurts to ask. I score some great deals this way.

***Pay attention to organic foods that aren't expensive to buy relative to conventional foods (bananas, for example).** Load up on those.

***Be smart when picking what you buy as organic.** Some conventionally grown foods have higher levels of pesticides than others. For those, go organic. Then, for foods that aren't sprayed as much, consider conventional. Avocados, for example, aren't sprayed too much, so you could buy those as conventional. Check out Environmental Working Group's Shopper's Guide to Pesticides at FoodNews.org/walletguide.php for a handy list (I also recommend their iPhone app).

***Buy food on sale.** Produce prices vary a lot based on supply. Pay attention to which organic foods are on sale and plan your week's menu around those. These savings can really add up!

***Grow your own sprouts.** They are very inexpensive, and it's much easier than it sounds. Sprouts are really healthful due to their high concentration of nutrients and ease of digestion. Load up on these for salads, soups, and smoothies. Buy organic seeds in the bulk bins at your natural foods store, or buy online and grow them yourself. This is fun for kids—they love to watch them grow!

***Buy organic seeds and nuts in bulk online and freeze them.** Nuts and seeds are less expensive when you order in bulk from sites like BlueMountainOrganics.com. Frozen nuts and seeds will last an entire year, so stock up. For certain items, like almonds, I buy 30 pounds (14 kg) at a time! My mom buys small portions from me and I freeze the rest. I also buy hemp seeds in bulk—a 25-pound (11-kg) bucket. These foods make great gifts, too. Buy in bulk, save money, and then give away a mason jar of almonds or hemp seeds (or whatever food you bought in bulk) tied with a bow as a gift during the holidays. Stock up on dried fruits, too.

Another money-saving tip: When making a recipe that calls for nuts, you can often replace them with less-expensive options like sunflower seeds or pumpkin seeds. I also use raisins instead of dates sometimes for the same reason.

***Buy seasonally.** For instance, don't buy raspberries in December. Not only do they cost a lot, but they're also probably from Mexico or South America, which enlarges your carbon footprint. Consider buying frozen organic fruits as well, especially when they're on sale. As with all produce, if you pay attention to prices for a while, you'll naturally start taking advantage of price dips.

***Shop at your farmers' markets or join a CSA for the best prices and to get really local with your produce.** This is the best way!

As a recap, it is essential to use organic ingredients for many reasons:

***The health benefits.** Superior nutrition, reduced consumption of chemicals and heavy metals, and decreased exposure to carcinogens. Studies have shown that some organic foods have up to 300 percent more nutrition than conventionally grown produce. And a very important note for pregnant women: pesticides can cross the placenta and affect the fetus. Make organics an extra priority if you're pregnant.

***Better taste.** I've had people tell me in my raw food demonstration classes that they never knew vegetables tasted so good.

***Greater variety.** Heirloom fruits and vegetables are the result of organic farming.

***Ecology.** Buying organic means cleaner rivers and waterways for Earth and its inhabitants, along with minimized erosion of topsoil. Organic farming builds up the soil better, reduces carbon dioxide in the air, and can help make life on the planet sustainable for generations to come.

CHAPTER 5

EXPECTATIONS

Great things happen when you go raw. You will quickly experience weight loss, increased energy, soft skin, clear eyes, silky hair, better sleep, mental clarity, major health improvements, a peaceful mind-set, and more.

LABELS AND YOUR RAW FOOD "IDENTITY"

Another thing you can expect is that as soon as friends and family members learn that you're "into raw food," they'll probably have questions. As with questions about veganism and vegetarianism, many people's questions implicitly try to categorize you neatly into one camp or another with "Do you eat this?" and "Do you eat that?" type questions. I find that the real-world practice of eating raw is much less tidy than that. For every "yes" or "no" I give, I might have quite a few "maybe's" and "it depends."

There are different raw food camps when it comes to which plan is the best, which "version" of raw, if you will. While all raw fooders agree on the benefits of eating raw, they debate some of the details, sometimes down to splitting hairs. This leads to contradictory advice that can be confusing for beginners, as it was for me when I first started. (It doesn't help matters that the scientific research on raw food is woefully lacking, though it is improving all the time.)

People also vary in terms of degree. Those on the extreme end of the raw food spectrum lead a very strict lifestyle, eating almost exclusively raw. Some of them don't even use salt, garlic, or ginger in their food because they believe these foods are too stimulating. Next on the raw spectrum are the "high raw" people discussed earlier, who eat anywhere from 75 to 99 percent of their diet raw. And then there is the broadest group of raw fooders, people who just generally try to fit more raw food into their diets when possible (such as 50 to 75 percent of their food intake).

In short, eating "raw" is a matter of degree, and the label means different things to different people. I think that labels are limiting when they pigeonhole us into an unnecessarily narrow set of options. Living a raw food lifestyle is an evolutionary process. Rather than worrying about labels and rules, a better approach is to experiment, keep trying new things, and find what works best for you without worrying about how to describe your lifestyle. And then expect it to continuously evolve over time.

The approach you take will depend on your goals and where you are on your personal journey. If your lifestyle recently included eating lots of sugary cooked desserts, then a raw dessert sweetened with raw agave nectar will be a dramatic improvement. On the other hand, if you are already eating pretty cleanly or watching your weight, you might find yourself avoiding desserts altogether, whether they're raw or not. I always say, "Listen to your body," because that way you'll figure out what makes you feel best. Fine-tune things as you go, taking it one day at a time, and having fun with the ongoing process of discovery.

There are a lot of books available with different opinions about raw food. Except for being strictly vegan, I don't follow any one program all the way. Everyone is different and might react differently to certain foods. However, there is one common denominator and great rule of thumb: the more raw plant-based foods people eat, the better they tend to feel. After that, no single detail is worth getting too worked up about. Just take it all in and try to see the big picture. The most important thing is to begin. Try new ways of eating, resist old unhealthful habits, and see raw food for what it is: a fun and fascinating way to explore a whole new world. Start today.

One of the most tragic things I know about human nature is that all of us tend to put off living. We are all dreaming of some magical rose garden over the horizon instead of enjoying the roses blooming outside our windows today.
—Dale Carnegie

DETOXIFICATION

Detoxification is the process whereby the body eliminates toxins that have been accumulating over long periods of time. Very often, when you stop ingesting new toxins by converting to a cleaner, toxin-free diet, your body seizes the opportunity to clean house of all of the garbage that it has been accumulating. In the informal lingo of nutrition, this unpleasant but good-for-you process is known as "detoxing."

It is not unlikely that you'll experience detox in some form when you start eating a diet that is high in fresh raw food, especially if your dietary shift is dramatic and fast. The best thing you can do is to be prepared mentally, knowing in advance that the experience is not permanent. Part of being prepared is knowing what to expect. Detox varies for people, based on their existing dietary habits, individual history, behaviors, age, environment, and genes. Your experience will differ from another's because of what toxins you might already have in you, plus your current lifestyle.

What to Expect During Detox

After a period of time, the body builds up toxins and natural waste products from chemicals, pollution, and foods that are difficult for the body to break down. A process of cleansing the internal system, or "detoxifying," helps to rid the body of harmful chemicals that may be contributing to fatigue, illness, pain, and poor digestion. When you remove toxin-laden foods from your diet, the body's resources are freed to remove toxins that have been building up in the body, often for many years.

During detoxification, the body eliminates these built-up toxins the same way it always does, through the eliminative organs: the skin, bowels, urinary tract, etc. Shifting to a vegan and/or raw diet therefore is often initially accompanied by cold- or allergy-like symptoms, particularly the production of phlegm. This is temporary, and can be a satisfying experience once you realize that the mucus your body is expelling is literally garbage that you have been carrying around in your tissues for a long time. And once it's out, it's out, leaving your cleansed body in a much healthier, cleaner, efficient state.

Some people experience bloating, skin eruptions, headaches, body aches, a runny nose, extreme fatigue, mood swings and flaring emotions, weight loss, and more when going through detoxification from a raw diet. Don't be surprised if you experience any of these symptoms.

One of my favorite experiences when going raw was the detox period. Yes, this process can be painful for some people. It was no picnic for me, either. I had headaches, pain, a snotty nose, skin rashes, and horrible tiny pimples—my face suddenly looked like sandpaper with all the little bumps. I thought, “Where did these come from?” I instinctively knew it was the detox, and I felt relief to know that toxins were leaving my body. It was scary, too, as I realized I'd been carrying those toxins around inside of me for a long time. It was liberating and worth it. I wish I had taken photos of my detox symptoms as a reminder of what not to eat when I am craving something unhealthful. The length of detox is based on a variety of factors: how healthy your eating was before, your age, etc. Basically, the earlier you start, the easier it will be!

Here are some things that you might try to help ease the pain if you have headaches while detoxing:

* Acupressure: Firmly (until it's slightly uncomfortable) pinch the tendons deep in the meaty part of the V between your thumb and index finger. Do this on each hand or have someone do it for you. This releases endorphins in the brain. You'll often start to feel the headache go away within a minute or two.
* Drink warm herbal tea.
* Take a warm bath with the lights turned low, in total silence or with soft music playing.
* Get a foot rub and/or a massage.
* Rub your temples and/or eyebrows with gentle pressure.
* Stretch and breathe deeply.
* Drink fresh, alkalizing green juice.

WEIGHT LOSS

I feel the healthiest, sexiest, and most energetic when I'm not carrying around extra weight. I've tried almost every diet, but I never once succeeded with healthy, long-term, feel-good weight loss—until I went raw. Losing weight by any other than a plant-based diet is generally the result of bodily distress (more stress on the kidneys), meaning that it's probably not for the long term and you will gain the weight back. And, if it is for the long term, your body may pay a heavy price for it later, because you've stressed it in such an unhealthy way.

The American Cancer Society conducted a study over a ten-year period with eighty thousand people trying to lose weight. The participants who ate meat three times a week gained substantially more weight than those who didn't and ate more vegetables instead. Another study published in the *New England Journal of Medicine* stated that meat eaters are much more likely to be overweight than vegetarians. Eating meat is not the answer to losing weight. (Atkins results, for example, are generally temporary, and according to Brian Wansink, author of *Mindless Eating*, similar weight loss can be seen in any diet that limits what you eat to any one food—say, corn—because your body naturally gets tired of eating just one food and you stop eating. All such diets are unhealthy, because no one food provides adequate nutrition.)

One of the reasons that weight loss happens so easily with a raw food diet has to do with how the food is assimilated and digested in your body. Many people who always feel hungry do so because they are not getting the proper nutrition their body needs. If you find yourself hungry all the time, as I used to, that's because your body is crying out for nutrients. Listen to your body! Almost all vitamins and nutrients can be found in fresh raw food. And, because raw food has its nutrients intact, your body can properly assimilate them. When this happens, your hunger tends to decrease.

I used to be a big food worshipper with an over-the-top appetite. I would boast to my male friends that I could "out-eat" them—not a feminine challenge, I know. At buffets I would bring back two to three plates in one trip, and I would use a dinner plate for the dessert table. I used to be so consumed by food that it was not uncommon for me to think about what I was going to eat for lunch when it was only breakfast, as well as eagerly anticipating dinner before my lunch had even started. I was obsessed with food.

Since going raw, my appetite has reduced, and I don't obsess about my meals far in advance. In the beginning stages, when I was transitioning from cooked to raw (and the same thing may happen to you), I continued to eat the same quantity of food. At that point, the struggle was more of a mental game than a physical hunger. When you say good-bye to something in your life, it can be a tough transition for your mind, so take your time doing this and enjoy the journey.

Raw can seem like a huge change, and indeed it is if you go 100 percent raw all at once. But you don't have to go 100 percent raw in the beginning (or maybe ever, for that matter) to see amazing results. Just start eating "more" raw foods and listen to your body as you go. You're not only putting great food into your body, you'll also stop eating all kinds of garbage, such as cholesterol, trans fats, and processed sugars. And you'll start feeling better and better and better.

Eating raw is a completely new approach to food, lifestyle, and health. It's not about counting calories, which will be a welcome relief to many people who want to lose weight. All you have to do is eat raw foods, as much as you want, within reason. There are no formulas to memorize or carry around with you, no rules about which foods to eat or at which times of day. A raw food diet is about feeling alive as your body works wonders, and experiencing, perhaps for the first time in your life, what it feels like to be firing on all cylinders.

Are You Still Hungry?

Some people are eager to lose weight as quickly as possible. If this is you, here are a few tips to help:

***Eat apples. Apples tend to fill you up quickly and sufficiently because of their pectin.** Sometimes I eat an apple about twenty minutes before a meal. This helps me to eat less at the meal.

***Drink a fresh green smoothie.** This does the trick every time! If you can't make a smoothie, then grab a piece of fruit.

***Drink warm organic miso soup.** My favorite brand is South River Miso (available at SouthRiverMiso.com). They offer both soy and non-soy varieties.

***Drink organic herbal tea (ginger or peppermint are my favorites).** If you like your tea sweet, add a little raw agave nectar or stevia. There is something satiating about these teas that really helps to "take the edge off."

***Brush your teeth.** This often seems to curb the appetite. As a reminder, keep a toothbrush with some all-natural toothpaste with you at all times.

***Take a ten-minute walk.** I find that taking a quick walk can curb my appetite for a while and refresh me at the same time.

***Drink a raw protein shake using a protein powder.** This can help you feel full right away. I'm a fan of both organic hemp protein powder as well as sprouted brown rice protein powder. Try a quick shake made from water and 1 to 2 scoops of Sun Warrior's sprouted raw vegan brown rice protein powder (I prefer the chocolate flavor and like to add ¼ teaspoon or more of cinnamon and a dash of nutmeg). Another great brand to try is Sprout Living. Details for these products are available at KristensRaw.com/store.

ENERGY

Get ready for some explosive energy when you start living the raw food lifestyle. Having excellent digestion, proper nutrition, and peaceful sleep all contribute to giving you skyrocketing energy that lasts all day long. There's a good chance that you'll sleep less, too, meaning you can get more done in your day. Who doesn't want that?

Most Americans consume too much protein, and this is one of the main reasons people feel sluggish and tired. Animal protein is an energy drainer, because it's hard for your body to digest. Dr. Andrew Weil states that when his patients come to him with lack of energy, one of the first recommendations he gives is to reduce their consumption of animal protein.

Another reason Americans are tired is from coming off the highs of caffeine, which causes exhaustion. Before I went raw and vegan, I was a victim of both too much protein and adrenal exhaustion from all the caffeine and other stimulants (like the over-the-counter body-enhancing pills used for my body-building) I was consuming. My lack of energy was, in fact, one of the driving forces behind my search for healthier living. I was tired of being tired. To try to give myself energy, I was drinking two to three triple-espresso soy cappuccinos daily. I knew this was unhealthy, and it scared me.

Now, I have energy that lasts all day. I wake up naturally, without my alarm clock, ready to take on the day. I don't need caffeine to get my brain functioning, because I'm not groggy when I wake up. I'm focused and alert. It's a wonderful feeling.

The difference between one man and another is not mere ability, it is energy.
—Thomas Arnold

DIGESTION

Digestion Timeline

There are 100 million nerves in your intestines. This is not a body part you want to clog up or coat with toxic sludge. After you eat a meal, blood is shunted to your digestive system and away from your muscles, brain, and other organs. This is the reason people often feel like resting after eating a big cooked meal instead of going out for a jog.

When cooked food is in your system too long, it can ferment and putrefy, causing indigestion, heartburn, and weight gain. In contrast, fruits and vegetables, which are mostly water, take only a short time to travel through the digestive tract. I never feel as if I have to "recover" after eating raw food, the way I did when I ate cooked food.

Here's just one example of the time needed to get cooked animal food versus fresh raw plant food through your digestive system.

* **Steak:** Two to three days (during which it basically starts to rot)

* **Raw fruit and vegetables:** Less than twelve hours!

Pooping: A Direct Link to Your Health

While we're on the topic of digestion and elimination, let's talk about poop. Here is a good rule of thumb: You should be sitting on the porcelain throne to poop about the same number of times as you eat in a day. Yes, you read that correctly! If you're eating three to four meals a day, you should poop three to four times a day as well. It varies a little for each person depending on how you combine your food, how much liquid you are consuming, and so on, but this gives you an idea. Now, when I tell people this in my classes, I usually see some jaws drop. All this time they considered themselves lucky to poop once a day! If you've been eating the Standard American Diet for a long time, you will probably have so much poop and waste backed up in your body that it could take many trips to the toilet before you get with a regular routine. But once things get regular, the poops get very healthy—fast, efficient, and easy. On a raw diet, you may never be constipated again!

One last note on the subject of healthy poops: It may come as a surprise that most of the world poops in a squatting position rather than sitting. As a result, hemorrhoids are far less common in countries where squatting is the norm. It makes sense when you think about it: our digestive systems evolved in a world that had no toilets, and everybody squatted. This posture makes for a more direct elimination path and less straining. Fortunately, to take advantage of this, you don't need to move to Thailand or retrofit the plumbing fixtures in your house. All you need is a simple wooden device called a Miracle Step, which fits at the base of any household toilet. Just squat on the Miracle Step when you're doing your business and feel what nature intended all along. We have one in our house and we love it! (For more information, visit KristensRaw.com/store.)

Things to Help Your Digestion—Today

The following are some tips to help your digestion so you can start feeling better immediately. You will find that these not only aid in digestion, but also help prevent gas and abdominal discomfort.

* **Chew your food to a mush.** This converts food to a consistency that's almost liquid, which helps save your body's energy when digesting the food chemically farther downstream. I know, we all heard it when we were kids, "Chew your food!" But it's true, so pay attention and make sure you're actually doing it. I always used to forget; the only way I was able to make it a permanent habit was to write on a sticky note "CHEW FOOD TO A MUSH" and put it anyplace where I ate (dining room table, desk, night stand, kitchen counter). It worked. It only took about two weeks of having those sticky notes around until it became a habit. After that, I was able to discard the notes and the habit stuck.

* **Do not drink liquids within a half hour prior to eating food or an hour after your meal.** This might seem counterintuitive. Sometimes people who want to lose weight are advised to drink a big glass of water right before a meal to help "fill them up" so they will eat less. But we now know that this actually impedes digestion. When you drink liquids, you dilute your own natural digestive juices, which makes it harder for your body to digest food.

* **Soak raw nuts and seeds before eating them.** This is important for optimal digestion. It's not required, but recommended. See page 80 for more details.

* **Eat melons without other foods.** This will speed the digestion of the melon and prevent it from starting to ferment in your digestive tract. There are a number of food-combining principles (see page 126) that can help digestion, but this is the one I follow religiously to avoid feeling bloated. Watermelon, cantaloupe, honeydew melons, and other melons should not be eaten within 25 to 30 minutes of eating other foods or within four hours after eating high-fat or high-protein foods. The ideal time to eat melon is first thing in the morning, after you've spent the night sleeping (naturally fasting).

CHAPTER 6

A DAY IN THE LIFE OF RAW

What does a typical raw food day look like? While this varies for everyone, depending on individual goals, there are some common elements. One of the things I love about the raw food diet is that it can be followed by anyone to some degree and at any stage of life and it will yield immediate beneficial results. This is a lifestyle that people all around the world have adopted and stayed on for decades because they experience true health as never before. People love living the raw lifestyle because it works. Once you do it, you always want to do it at some level. Your eating patterns will forever be changed. You'll feel better emotionally, physically, mentally, and spiritually, and that is addictive, my friend.

Raw food can work for you whether you are short on time or whether you have ample occasion every week to prepare food. I easily make it work for me, no matter what's going on in my life. When I'm on the go, I grab fresh, crisp apples or bananas for breakfast, or I blend up a fast smoothie. When I have more time for food preparation, I make crunchy and sweet raw granola with fresh almond milk and strawberries. The wonderful thing about a raw food diet is that it can be simple, easy, varied, and still full of flavor.

Keep in mind that baby steps and incremental improvements in your diet will bring benefits. Don't feel pressured to start 100 percent raw tomorrow, although you might want to. In fact, that plan does work for many people, but when they do it, they usually spend some time beforehand preparing. They stock their kitchens with the right foods and equipment. If necessary, they explain their plan to their loved ones. Some people even plan the different foods they want to make for the first two to four weeks. Essentially, they strategize what they need to do to succeed. When you plan ahead and jump in guns a-blazin', success can be yours. However, there is no shame in taking it slowly. Instead of jumping in with both feet, you can put in one toe at a time. For many people, a gradual approach is ideal.

BREAKFAST

Here are some examples for energizing raw breakfasts. Sometimes, I simply eat fresh fruit. For example, I'll eat a couple of bananas or apples. A nice breakfast fruit salad is diced apple, mango, and avocado. Squirt a little fresh lime on top. Yum! I'm also a fan of green smoothies and green juice (which I like to call Plant Blood because it makes me feel badass). With smoothies, you can make a giant batch at once, then store it in the fridge and drink it over the next two to three days. I use mason jars, filled almost to the top with smoothie so there's as little air in there as possible, which helps keep the liquid from oxidizing. Raw granola with raw nut milk is a treat (you can make raw granola, see page 148, or buy it premade from a natural foods store or online). And sometimes, I even eat a raw dessert, such as Date Bars (page 189) or Sweet Chia Pudding (page 186) for breakfast. Why not? It's healthful!

LUNCH

Lunch offers many delicious options. I might eat a giant vegetable salad with a fantastic raw dressing that makes me want to lick the bowl clean. Other times I drink a big green smoothie or eat a satiating raw soup with some flax crackers and raw cheese spread or raw hummus—absolutely divine.

Soups and smoothies are fantastic for your digestive system, and they can give you extra energy because your body doesn't have to work nearly as hard breaking down food that's already in liquid form. They are also a great way to eat more greens, so you are getting filled with healthful body- and bone-building minerals. When I make a soup for my lunch, I make a large batch that lasts two to three days. For added variation with the soup, on the last day, I might use it as a sauce on zucchini pasta or kelp noodles, or I might water it down (if needed) and use it as a dressing on a big salad of chopped vegetables. Food has never been so easy, simple, delicious, and nutritious.

ENTREES

Dinner is a special time for eating because this is usually when we sit down with family. There are many options, from simple entrees such as nut pâté stuffed in fresh red bell peppers to garden burgers to zucchini pasta marinara to more gourmet options like raw pizza, lasagna, or quiche. You'll find that you and your family are eating the most satisfying, healthful, and delicious food imaginable. Some dishes take more time to prepare; others are amazingly fast, and with raw food, cleanup is always a snap because there's no cooked-on food or grease to deal with. You might never touch a scouring pad again!

DESSERTS

Almost every dessert you'd normally cook, you can make raw—in fact, it's usually easier. Raw cobblers, cookies, pies, brownies, mousses, ice creams, and cheesecakes are just a few of the delights that await you.

I don't know many people who do not like desserts. There might be people who don't eat them, but it's not usually because they don't like them (think skinny supermodels). Well, I have excellent news for both you and them (the skinny models, that is). The greatest thing about raw desserts is that they appeal to everyone (including non-vegans and non-raw-fooders, including the world's most brutal critics: kids and your mother-in-law).

Raw desserts can be eaten any time of the day because they are healthful, especially when compared to a standard cooked dessert that's loaded with refined sugar. Raw desserts are much healthier than the normal breakfast foods that most people eat (scones, muffins, high-sugar cereals with cow's milk, buttered toast—and don't even get me started on the heart-gunking insanity that is bacon and eggs!). Sometimes you'll find me eating a raw chocolate cookie—for breakfast.

Because mousses and puddings freeze well, I usually store them in 1-cup (240-ml) mason jars. This way, I can take out a small jar for a couple of days while keeping the rest of it frozen if I'm the only one eating it. The same goes for raw cheesecake. I slice the part I'm not eating right away and freeze the slices individually to enjoy at a later date. You should see my freezer. We could eat for weeks with what's typically stored in there. I find that having this much food on hand, ready to eat at any time, makes my life simpler and allows more flexibility and spontaneity in other aspects of life.

MY FOOD JOURNAL

The readers of my blog are always asking to see raw food meal plans or wanting to know what I eat in a typical day. Through their feedback, comments, questions, and suggestions, I've been trained to mention my daily menu frequently—with all of the variety available, it never gets old.

For this reason, I have a Food Journal link on my blog where you can see many days of what it's like to eat all raw and high raw; just visit KristensRaw.com/blog. People tell me that this ongoing food journal and other readers' comments help to keep them motivated and on track. It's wonderful to be part of an online community of like-minded people!

Things to Note About My Food Journal

Every morning, when I wake up, I drink about 8 ounces (240 ml) of water. I find that I do this most consistently if I put a glass bottle of water on my nightstand at bedtime so that it's ready for me in the morning. This is great for cleansing the body and perfect for helping you "get going" in the morning when it comes to pooping.

Fresh vegetable juice (a.k.a. green juice, a.k.a. Plant Blood) is a staple in my life for optimal health. This is where I get loads of vitamins, minerals, phytonutrients, and enzymes in the most easily absorbed form. As Normal Walker writes in *Fresh Vegetable and Fruit Juices*, "Any person not familiar with the nutritional and recuperative value of fresh vegetable and fruit juices is woefully uninformed." My usual routine is to drink 16 to 32 ounces (480 to 960 ml) of fresh veggie juice after I'm up and about in the morning (I don't always do this daily, but pretty close). My juice recipes vary, but the ones I especially enjoy include cucumber, zucchini, and celery. These make up the base, and then I add a hearty green such as kale, collard greens, broccoli, or Swiss chard, depending on whether I'm in the mood for smooth 'n' mellow or Yowza Holy Green, Batman! Finally, a lovely squeeze of citrus rounds it out.

During the day, I usually have a big salad. When I say a big salad, I'm not kidding—I mean a *big* salad. I'm not shy on the amount of lettuce and veggies because I want it to fill me up. I usually top it off with 2 to 4 tablespoons of raw dressing. I usually water down the dressing a little so it spreads easily over most of the lettuce and veggies. This helps to add flavor but not a lot of extra calories from fat. Another trick is to use salad tongs to toss the salad well so it's evenly coated. When I do this, I find that I need less dressing to achieve complete coverage.

In my journal, you may notice that I don't have my foods portioned out as breakfast, lunch, or dinner. That's because I tend to graze all day. So, if you see foods listed with no spacing between them, then I ate them at the same sitting. Once you see a space between line items, that means there was at least an hour between foods.

Following is a brief sample of my online Food Journal posts:

A Typical High-Raw Day

* Protein shake made with Sun Warrior protein powder and homemade curry powder
* Grapefruit
* Kombucha
* Six-Minute Lasagna Stack
* 2 small apples
* Black beans (cooked) with fresh guacamole, fresh salsa, and chopped romaine lettuce (In a high-raw diet, cooked legumes are fine; in an all-raw diet, you can sprout many legumes instead of cooking them.)
* Five-Minute Walnut-Oatmeal Brownies with a glass of cold Brazil nut milk
* 1 banana
* 1 grapefruit

A Typical All-Raw Day

* 3 cups (720 ml) lemon-lime broccoli juice
* Sun Warrior protein shake
* 2 cups (480 ml) vitamin C green smoothie
* Spiced Apricot-Date Granola with raw Brazil nut milk
* Coleslaw
* Cheezy Hemp Nacho Kale Chips
* Collard All-Star Wrap
* Citrus-Cauliflower Soup
* 2 chocolate nut butter balls

As you can see, I get *plenty* of variety on a raw food diet. People who are afraid that a raw lifestyle would be a rabbit-like existence of nibbling on carrot sticks and lettuce all day long have no idea what amazing food awaits them!

CHAPTER 7

WHERE ARE YOU TODAY?

Everyone knows that they should be eating more fruits and vegetables, right? It's no secret that most people need more fresh whole foods in their diet. With raw cuisine, it's never been easier. Or more exciting! I promise that you will look forward to your raw fruits and vegetables (as never before), because they taste great and are prepared in amazing new ways that even world-class celebrity chefs on your favorite TV shows aren't familiar with—not yet, anyway.

Your first step on the path to raw food is to identify where you are now in your dietary habits and lifestyle, and then use the following information to figure out the next steps that are right for you. See what makes the most sense, and as you dive in, what makes you feel the healthiest and go from there.

The first thing to remember is, don't limit your options by strictly defining how much raw food you intend to eat. Stay flexible. Just eat what you need and what seems natural. Your body will guide you. This is super important to ensure your success, so you don't feel deprived. A sense of deprivation is one of the biggest reasons people fail on any diet. When I first went raw, in only a short period of time I had fewer and fewer cravings until I was completely satisfied with my new lifestyle. Think about that. I never missed the unhealthful foods I had eliminated from my diet. It didn't take discipline—I just liked what I was doing. You can do exactly the same thing. And at the risk of sounding like a broken record, you must remain flexible in order to have nutritional variety. I have days where I want only fruits and vegetables, and other days when I want nut pâtés and desserts. And then I switch back again. Or I go crazy on some new recipe for a week and then don't eat it again for six months. Seriously, I never know where raw food is going to lead me, and I love that. This way of life is an exciting evolution, so embrace it, enjoy it, and take it one day, week, or month at a time. Be flexible, keep making adjustments, and listen to your body.

The next step is to reduce or eliminate unhealthful food from your diet. This includes junk food, packaged and processed snacks, animal-based products, fried foods, all white sugar, and all white flour. Here is the fun part: Go through your cabinets and throw these junk foods away. Don't say, "I'll just eat the rest of these so I don't waste them." No! Throw that junk out! Ceremoniously, if you like. Your life is changing. You are on a new path to optimal health. When I did this, I cranked up the soundtrack from *Rocky III* and filled my ears with "Eye of the Tiger," and it totally pumped me up. I threw that junk food into the trash with ferocity (because it was "junk" after all!). Then, I took a picture of the garbage in my trash can so I would remember it as that—garbage.

PLAN OF ATTACK

One option is to go cold turkey. This was not something I wanted to do, because I had to get off caffeine, which was a gradual process in my case. If you're inspired to go cold turkey, great. There's no right or wrong way to go raw.

Another option is having a nice transition to the raw lifestyle. When taking this approach, you can do it one of two ways: Divide the day into raw meals and non-raw meals. This means that maybe you'll have a raw breakfast and raw lunch but a cooked vegan dinner. Or, divide each meal into raw food and cooked food, gradually increasing the percentage of raw food on the plate.

The other option is to have certain days of the week when you eat 100 percent raw and other days when you eat part raw and part cooked vegan. This method worked best for me, so I'll go into detail with that plan.

IF YOU ARE NEW TO RAW . . .

Start out by picking one day a week (or more, if you want) to eat 100 percent raw all day long. You'll see how easy it is and how amazing you feel. You'll soon be excited to do more than one day a week, maybe two or three days. After that, start increasing to one week straight, then two weeks, then up to a month (leaving a little wiggle room here and there, for times when you can't do it, perhaps due to social situations). Find what works for you.

It's important to write your plan for going raw on your calendar. Planning it and putting it in writing is one the best ways to help you accomplish your goal so you don't get off track. I put sticky notes on the fridge and kitchen cabinets, and sometimes I even write in dry-erase marker on the mirror in my dressing area.

On the days you're 100 percent raw, write "Today is 100% Raw—no exceptions." On the days that your goal is not to be 100 percent raw, simply start adding more raw foods to your daily food choices. For example, you might commit to three days of 100 percent raw and four days of 50 percent raw (don't let the other 50 percent cooked be junk or processed foods though—pick something that is still relatively healthful—and be sure to stay vegan, no exceptions).

Some people follow this plan by eating a salad before lunch and dinner or having their traditional cooked vegetable side dishes made from raw food instead (and then having only the main course be cooked). Or, some people start by having a piece of fruit before their normal cooked breakfast. Another option is to have a cooked dinner, but have a raw breakfast and lunch on the days that you are not 100 percent raw.

Remember, if you fall off the wagon, don't worry, just get right back on. Every minute of every day is a chance to make your body and soul healthier. Take advantage of it!

EATING ARTFULLY, GLAMOROUSLY, AND HEALTHFULLY

We feast with our eyes first because we look at what we eat before we eat it. If something looks good, then we are predisposed to think it tastes good. Appearance really does influence how food tastes. This is where raw food is especially easy, because it's full of beautiful, radiant, and vibrant colors from healthful phytonutrients. "A rainbow a day" in my food is what I aim to accomplish.

To take your meals to the next level of enjoyment, make your eating experience the best ever with the help of a simple, gorgeous, and glamorous presentation. I use my best dishes when I eat. I use beautiful wineglasses for my smoothies and juices. I use fancy goblets for many of my desserts. Why? Because I'm worth it (and so are you!). Nothing makes plain water taste better than sipping it from a sexy, beautiful wineglass. Don't save your good china for company only; indulge today, and every day. Believe me, you'll notice the difference. Your family will notice, too. Eating well is an attitude, and when you take care of yourself, your body, heart, and soul will respond in kind. It's like being on vacation at a luxurious resort every day of your life!

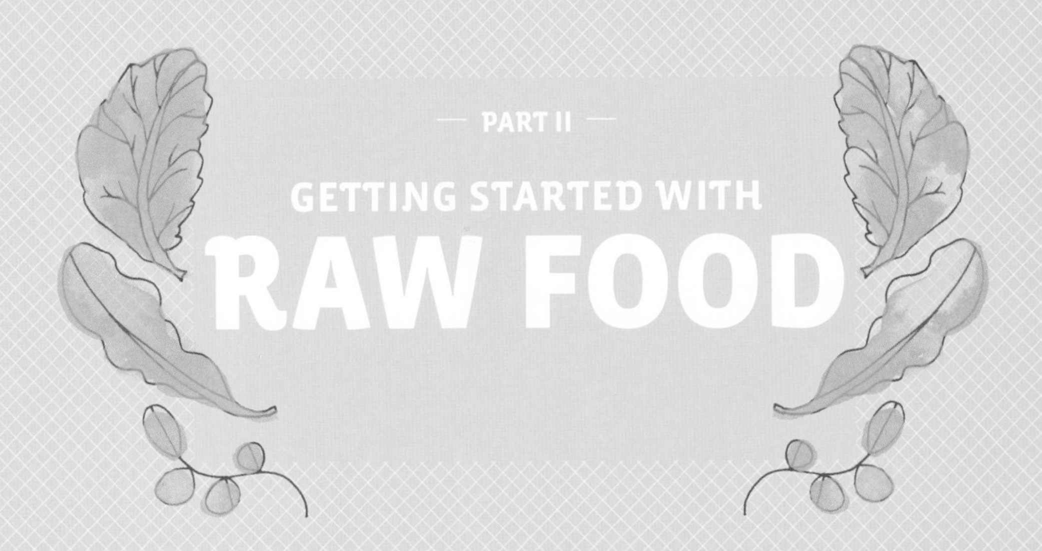

— PART II —

GETTING STARTED WITH RAW FOOD

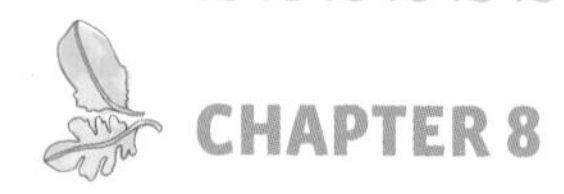

CHAPTER 8

EQUIPPING YOUR RAW FOOD KITCHEN

Isn't this exciting? There's more fun to come, because now I'll teach you about getting the proper equipment for your new raw food kitchen. It starts with freedom from the stove, oven, and microwave. And, oh what a freedom that is! In fact, my oven and microwave are both used for storage. My stove has a glass tabletop on top of it (from an old end table I no longer used), where I set all of my spices and seasonings. This way, they're always out and in sight for me to use. And I keep all of my equipment on my counter, so that it's ready for me to use and I don't forget about it. That way, every time I walk through my kitchen, I am reminded of my healthy raw lifestyle, and I feel proud and dedicated to have these great tools. They are also a fun conversation starter when people visit. My kitchen always intrigues people, and I love demonstrating the equipment for them so they can sample raw goodies right then and there. That's how I get them hooked! *Shhhhhh . . . don't tell.*

Here's a list of everything I recommend. The more you get, the easier raw food prep will be for you. However, as I've said before, baby steps are perfectly okay if that's how you'd prefer to proceed. So take your time transforming your kitchen and buy quality equipment that will last for years. Set yourself up for success and fun!

There are some other things to consider when plunking down a chunk of change for your kitchen equipment. Although good equipment can be pricey, it will also save you money. When you have a quality food processor, dehydrator, and blender, you can make your own raw staples such as nut butters, crackers, protein bars, and snacks. This can save a lot of money. You'll also eat out less, because you'll want to eat raw and there aren't a lot of raw food restaurants around, at least not yet. Not all the money for kitchen equipment has to come out of your own pocket. You can economize on equipment by building your kitchen with the help of others. When it comes to the holidays and your birthday, don't be shy about telling people exactly what you want, whether it's a shiny new juicer, a gift card to Amazon to go toward an appliance, or gift cards to Whole Foods Market. I've also redeemed credit card rewards for Amazon.com gift cards and used them to buy raw food appliances and supplies.

THE RAW FOOD KITCHEN

The following tools are listed in order of importance, beginning with what I consider essentials and then going on to items that you might want to add to your raw food kitchen as you go on with this lifestyle (the list includes many tools you might already have, so check them off if you do). The most preferred and recommended brands listed here (and some video reviews) can be found online via links on my Web site, KristensRaw.com/store.

Chef's knife and knife sharpener: The technique you will be using the most when prepping raw food is—chopping. Get a fantastic chef's knife. I cannot emphasize this enough. The brand I prefer and use at home is MAC. A great place to start is a knife that is 6 to 8 inches (15 to 20 cm) in length. Along with this, get an inexpensive knife sharpener. After you sharpen your knife, do the paper test on it. Hold up a piece of paper in one hand and see if your knife can cut it from top to bottom with ease. Be careful, of course.

Paring knife: An essential tool for small work.

Ceramic knives: Ceramic knives are unique in that they reduce oxidation of the foods you cut. They are extremely sharp and almost never need sharpening. They are fragile, though, so you have to be extra careful with them. That being said, they really rock! They are razor sharp and make you feel like you're cutting room-temperature butter with almost anything you cut. I do not use my ceramic knives on hard root vegetables because of the knives' fragility; instead I use them to cut leafy greens, fruit, soft vegetables, and herbs.

Blender (preferably high-powered): I use my blender multiple times a day—it's that important. I make smoothies, nut milks, ice creams, soups, mousses, and much more with it. When you are starting out, you can use any ol' blender. But as you start making more raw foods with nuts and seeds, it is helpful to have a high-powered blender. It's worth the money! I have both the Blendtec and Vita-Mix 5200 high-powered blenders. If I had to choose one, I'd probably go with the Vita-Mix 5200 (but they're both awesome—it's hard to decide). The Vita-Mix has a better warranty on both the container and base under normal household use (as of this writing). Check my Web site for more information on the two brands.

Food processor: Ideal for making crackers, pesto, ice cream, cookies, brownies, and much more. I also use my food processor rather than my blender to make nut butters, because it's easier to clean and easier to use. A 12- or 14-cup (2.5- or 3-L) processor is the best choice, because you will be able to make big batches of foods that last for a few days. I also highly recommend getting the extra discs when you can (1 mm, 2 mm, fine, shredding). I like both Cuisinart and KitchenAid brands.

Juicer: *"What kind of juicer should I get?"* This question is one of the most frequently asked by readers of my blog. The subject is a whole topic in itself because there is no one-size-fits-all answer. Every juicer has pros and cons, and the best one for you depends on your particular circumstances, lifestyle, and goals.

My personal obsession and ongoing quest to find the world's perfect juicer means that I have owned a lot of them over the years; in fact, I own three to four at any given time. (But don't worry, you'll do fine with just one.) Manufacturers are always introducing new models, too. This means that my recommendations about particular models change over time. For up-to-date video reviews of juicers, visit my blog at KristensRaw.com/juicers.

Juicing is important in the raw food diet, so you will need a good one. The key to obtaining juicing nirvana is to find the one that fits your lifestyle. The following guidelines will help you decide what's best for you.

The main things to consider are (1) price; (2) speed; (3) ease of cleanup; and (4) quality of the juice. Unfortunately, there is no one juicer that is inexpensive, fast, easy to clean, and makes very high-quality (non-oxidized) juice. The best you can hope for in a juicer is one that scores well in three of these four. (You can use a high-powered blender as a juicer if you strain the pulp, but this creates a lot of extra work. A juicer is a good investment if you plan to drink a lot of juice.)

If you're new to juicing, consider the Breville Ikon. It's lightning fast, easy to clean, and gives decent-quality juice for a reasonable price. (They also offer a smaller Breville that is less expensive but not quite as good due to its size and one-speed setting. It still does the job, though.)

If money and time are no objects, and you want very high-quality juice, then go for the Green Star. It's expensive and takes longer to juice, but its gears work in a way that avoids oxidation, making for extremely healthful juice. The Green Star juicer is high quality and will last years. (I've had mine for about seven years so far, and it still runs like new.)

A great happy medium between the lightning-fast Breville Ikon and the high-quality Green Star is the Hurom. If you're looking for quality juice that only takes a little more time to make than the Breville, then the Hurom is great. In many ways, it's the best of both worlds.

If you're going to be drinking a lot of juice (making yourself a true rawk star!), an important consideration is whether you'll be juicing multiple times per day versus juicing in bulk once and then drinking the juice throughout the day. If you'll be juicing multiple times, the Breville Ikon is a good choice due to its speed and convenience, and its lower-quality (more-oxidized) juice won't matter because you'll be drinking it immediately. But if you prefer to juice once and drink it throughout the day, then the Green Star's less-oxidized juice will keep better if stored in an airtight container in the fridge. Remember, the Green Star takes more time to clean, but you'll only be doing it once per day (or once every few days if you juice a really big batch—be sure to store juice in airtight glass containers filled to the top to reduce the exposure to oxygen).

Dehydrator: A dehydrator is basically a big box with a fan and a very low-heat heating element that, when run for hours, removes the moisture from food or warms it without actually cooking it, thereby preserving the food's raw nutritional value.

Many people are familiar with dehydrators for making dried fruit or fruit leather, but they don't know that dehydrators can be used for all kinds of other things, like making raw versions of breads, crackers, granola, snack bars, and for firming and concentrating foods like desserts and quiches. Plus, I am constantly using mine to dehydrate soaked nuts and seeds, thereby taking them back to a dry state but without the enzyme inhibitors intact (more on this in Chapter 9).

While not absolutely required for living a raw food lifestyle, dehydrators are important because they provide you with a ton of amazing raw food options. I use mine all the time. In fact, it's not often that you don't hear mine humming in our home.

In my opinion, Excalibur is by far the best manufacturer of consumer dehydrators. Their dehydrators come in five- and nine-tray varieties. I highly recommend going all out and buying the nine-tray model. Buying a large dehydrator—even though they don't cost much more—is making a commitment: "I'm going to do this." The food prep time (slicing fruit, for example, or spreading out a cracker mix) is not much more for large batches than small. And you don't run large dehydrators any longer than small dehydrators. So for basically the same amount of work, you get *much* more output from a large dehydrator. It's this higher output of delicious food per unit of effort that makes the nine-tray dehydrator an obvious choice for anybody who's interested in giving dehydrating a serious try. The nine-tray dehydrator is likely to become a permanent part of your routine; trust me, you'll use it. Whereas the five-tray is likely to become junk that you'll either never use after the first month or you'll try to get rid of when you decide to upgrade to a larger unit.

Make sure you also get the ParaFlexx nonstick sheets for each tray. These are made to fit the Excalibur brand, but you can use them in any dehydrator they fit into. You can use parchment paper in place of ParaFlexx sheets, but I find the ParaFlexx to be much more user-friendly. For some great tips on using your dehydrator, along with more recipes, see my book *Kristen Suzanne's EASY Raw Vegan Dehydrating*, available at KristensRaw.com.

Furthermore, I am happy to recommend Excalibur dehydrators because of their first-class products and customer service.

Proper Dehydration Techniques

When using a dehydrator, you'll usually want to begin the dehydrating process at a temperature of 130° to 140°F (54° to 60°C) for 1 to 2 hours. Then, lower the temperature to 105° to 110°F (40° to 43°C) for the remaining time of dehydration. Using a high temperature such as 140°F (60°C) *in the initial stages of dehydration* does not destroy the nutritional value of the food because, during this initial phase, the food does the most "sweating" (releasing moisture), which cools the food in the same way that sweat cools us when we exercise. Therefore, while the temperature of the air circulating *around* the food is about 140° F (60°C), the food itself is much cooler; in fact, it stays under the 118°F (48°C) mark that most raw fooders consider to still be "raw." (Note: These directions apply only when using an Excalibur Dehydrator, because of their Horizontal-Airflow Drying System.)

Spiral vegetable slicer: This amazing tool lets you spin food around an axis while a blade carves it up into fun spiral "noodles." Because you can use it to quickly and easily make vegetable pasta, it's considered by many to be a "must-have" for any raw food kitchen. If you have kids, then this is a must-have because kids love to use it (under adult supervision, of course), and gobbling up the veggie noodles becomes the highlight of their day! There are several different brands of this slicer, but my favorite is the Benriner Turning Slicer. It is more expensive than some others; however, the Benriner includes different blades to make different sizes of noodles, and the noodles have a better texture. The Benriner is higher quality, too (my other spiral slicer broke after a few years and I had to replace it, whereas my Benriner is still going strong after years of use).

The FoodSaver: Here is one of the best tips ever for raw food—Get a FoodSaver and make your life a million times easier with raw food prep. This is more than just a "food" saver, it's a life saver! For those who don't know, the FoodSaver is a vacuum suction device for storing food. It's a life saver because it dramatically improves the shelf life of raw food. I also use this nifty tool to magically accelerate the infusion process while marinating raw veggies. See Sous-Vide Veggies with Kelp Noodles (page 163).

You may know that FoodSavers suck the air out of special storage bags (which then get heat-sealed shut), but did you know that you can use a special attachment to vacuum-seal mason jars, too? This gives you a great way to store liquids. So when you think "FoodSaver" or vacuum-sealing, don't just think solids; think liquids, too (great for helping extend the life of your green juice).

When I make a soup that would normally last for three days, I use my FoodSaver and can now keep that same soup for up to a week (the FoodSaver people say it'll last much longer, but I always end up eating the food before I can see how long it actually does last). I do this with salad dressings, soups, desserts, fresh juices, smoothies, sauces, and much more. This is where the mason jar attachment comes in handy (you can find it at KristensRaw.com/store).

The FoodSaver is great for foods of all consistencies, from pesto to burgers to breads and crackers. I can't say enough about how fantastic this tool is in the kitchen. With the FoodSaver, you can make extra batches of foods and "FoodSaver" them so they last longer, meaning you can spend less time in the kitchen (I don't know if "to FoodSaver" is really a verb, but it definitely is in my kitchen!).

V-slicer (handheld) and/or mandoline: I recommend getting both a V-slicer (handheld model) and a mandoline. They are used for making thinly sliced foods (such as ravioli from beets). The mandoline is typically more expensive, but it ensures that you have very evenly sliced foods, it's much easier to control, and you can usually work faster with it. The mandoline is also ideal for larger quantities of foods. The V-slicer is great for foods when you don't care if they're perfectly and evenly sliced, and it's good for slicing small quantities. Mine gets frequent use for thinly slicing carrots and fennel to top my salads.

Travel blender: The real trick to successfully living the raw lifestyle is to stick with it even under less than ideal circumstances, such as when you're away from your awesomely equipped raw kitchen. Many people lose momentum on things like diet and exercise simply because they travel or have some other circumstance come up. But since we know these things happen in life, it's better to make plans than make excuses. Need to travel? No problem! Travel raw style. All it takes is a little preparation. I highly recommend buying a travel blender. In fact, it's a great tool to keep at your workplace, too: it's powerful, easy to clean, and portable. My favorite is the Tribest Personal Blender

(PB-100). I also use this to make baby food because it's great for small serving sizes.

Extra Gadgets to Have in Your Raw Kitchen

* Hand grater for shredding carrots or beets
* Fine zester/grater (Microplane)
* Bamboo cutting boards
* Hand citrus juicer
* Vegetable peeler
* Kitchen scissors
* Mason jars of various sizes (wide mouth)
* V-shaped dish rack for draining sprouts
* Bamboo sushi mat
* Vegetable scraper for the cutting board
* Garlic press
* Kitchen scale
* Wide-mouth funnel
* Cheesecloth
* Two to four colanders of different sizes
* Fine-mesh sieve
* Spreading spatulas (offset), large and small
* Rubber mixing spatulas of different sizes
* Springform pan(s) of different sizes (round and square)
* Spice (coffee) grinder
* Tart pan and pie dish
* Eight-inch (20-cm) square glass baking dish
* Salad spinner
* Two- and four-cup (500-ml and 1-L) liquid measuring cups
* Green produce bags (Evert Fresh)
* Two sets measuring spoons
* Two sets measuring cups
* One or two squeeze bottles for sauces
* Fruit scoopers (for avocados, mangos, and young Thai coconut)
* Salad tongs
* Mixing bowls
* Nut milk bags
* Lots of great serving dishes to present your food

CHAPTER 9

LET'S GO FOOD SHOPPING!

Although adopting the raw lifestyle might seem intimidating to some people, I'm here to show you that it can be easy. So, let's get to it. Consider the following options and pick the one that sounds right for you.

METHOD NO. 1: THE "GET ORGANIZED" PATH

This is a foolproof method to go raw, stay raw, and do it with gusto. It's all about *organization*. It was the way I originally started my raw lifestyle years ago. This path can be especially smart for raw newbies.

1. **Once a week, take your favorite raw recipe books and spend an hour flipping through them, salivating at all of the delicious options.** Decide what foods you want to make for the week and write your shopping list. It'll fast become something you look forward to doing every week.

2. **Schedule the recipes on your calendar so you know in advance what you're making on which days.** Keep in mind that if you're using nuts or seeds, you might need to soak or sprout them, so add those details to your calendar. For example, if you want to enjoy a recipe with soaked almonds on a Wednesday, then write on your calendar (or enter it into your smartphone) that you need to soak the nuts on Tuesday.

3. **Go shopping!**

METHOD NO. 2: THE "STAYING STOCKED" PATH

This path is great for the more seasoned raw foodie who is having trouble staying raw.

1. **Throw out the foods you don't want to be eating anymore.** Did they cost a lot? Too bad—just throw them out. Feel guilty about it? Don't. You're doing your body a favor.

2. **Stock your kitchen with all kinds of fresh produce and raw goodies.** You're not going by any kind of list. You're not checking recipes first. You're going to the store and buying a bunch of delicious produce, frozen fruits (if desired), dry essentials like nuts, seeds, agave nectar, cacao, dried fruits, seasonings, protein powders, and prepared raw snacks (crackers, cookies, etc.). See where your grocery cart takes you! Load up! Have fun! Buy in bulk!

So if you're a planning type of person, go with Method No. 1. If you like living on the edge and winging it, go with Method No. 2.

The second method is fun and exciting. I keep my kitchen loaded with various greens, fruits, vegetables, nut and seed butters, delicious spices, and more. Then, I make recipes based on whatever I have on hand, which is usually a little bit of everything. If I'm well stocked, there aren't too many recipes that I can't make. And, if there are one or two ingredients that I don't have, I can usually substitute something I have on hand. Using this method, I typically go to the store twice a week, so that my produce is always fresh and abundant in my kitchen. My counters are usually covered with bananas, mangoes, tomatoes, herbs, growing sprouts, apples, pears, and more. My refrigerator is literally *filled*—bursting at the seams—with greens, nut and seed butters, citrus, and more fruits and veggies. My kitchen just screams "raw food" everywhere I turn. It's a constant motivator and reminder about just how healthfully people can live if they decide to do so.

I love this style of "doing" raw, because it's great if my tastes change from one day to the next. I never know what mood I'll be in, but it doesn't matter because I have lots of options, and it's nearly impossible to fall off the path.

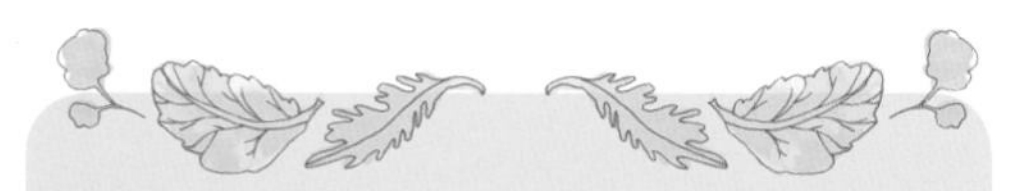

PRO TIP: For either of the strategies mentioned previously, I've found it's important to always have three things on hand in case of emergencies:

* 1 quart (960 mL) of raw vegan nut milk in the fridge
* Frozen peeled bananas in the freezer for soft-serve ice cream and shakes
* Packaged raw snacks in your cupboard, for when you don't have time to make your own

Don't these sound good? (Emergency rations like these make you look forward to emergencies!) I love Raw Almond Milk (page 177). I could drink this every day! Other staples in my kitchen are Pure Bars, Boku Bars, raw crackers, Blue Mountain Organics kale chips, trail mix, raw granola, nuts and seeds, dried fruit, raw protein powders, Rawtella (an amazing chocolate-hazelnut spread that I eat by the spoonful), and other delicious, satisfying snacks. It's impossible to not find something in my kitchen that tastes good, no matter what time of the day. And that is important for success!

Let's get to the nitty gritty now. In the following section, you will learn about stocking your raw kitchen, selecting and ripening produce, food storage, soaking and dehydrating nuts and seeds, and more.

STOCKING YOUR KITCHEN WITH RAW FOODS

In my kitchen, you'll find the following things. Keep in mind, I feed two people who eat high raw. I make a lot of green juices, smoothies, and salads, which account for much of the greens and fruit. I typically go to the store twice a week (or once a week and have food delivered once a week) to make sure I have these things on hand, plus an extra trip if necessary for special ingredients. You might not need all of the following items all of the time, but this list will give you an *idea* of what your refrigerator, counter, and pantry could look like. There are some foods (such as dates and tahini) that I don't buy every week because they last a while and I don't use them as regularly—but I always keep them stocked. Important note: unless they are unavailable, *all* items listed below should be organic.

Refrigerator

* Apple cider vinegar (keep in pantry until opened, then refrigerate)
* Apples
* Beets
* Carrots
* Cashew butter, almond butter, and tahini
* Celery
* Cucumbers (lots)
* Dried apricots
* Flax oil
* Fresh ginger
* Fresh herbs (such as parsley, cilantro, basil, dill, rosemary, and/or oregano)

* Hemp oil
* Kale (usually dark kale, also called dinosaur or lacinato, which is easier to wash and juice than curly kale)
* Lemons and/or limes
* Medjool dates
* Miso
* Mushrooms
* Nutritional yeast
* Olives
* Oranges
* Organic vegan white wine
* Probiotics powder or capsules
* Raisins
* Red cabbage
* Red, yellow, or orange bell peppers
* Romaine lettuce
* Seasonal fresh fruit
* Shallots
* Spinach
* Tamari, wheat-free
* Zucchini

Freezer

I have a separate free-standing freezer so that I can stock up on ingredients. It's worth the cost of the freezer and electricity because I save money when buying ingredients in bulk.

* Almonds, walnuts, pecans, pumpkin seeds, sunflower seeds, flaxseeds, sesame seeds, and chia seeds
* Bananas (peeled and stored in baggies or FoodSaver bags)
* Buckwheat groats
* Frozen corn (fresh corn that I buy in-season, shuck, and freeze)
* Frozen fruit
* Goji berries
* Raw carob
* Raw chocolate powder
* Raw oats
* Unsweetened shredded coconut

On the Counter

* Avocados
* Bananas (in varying stages of the ripening process)
* Garlic
* Growing sprouts (alfalfa, mung, clover, broccoli sprouts) in mason jars
* Organic vegan red wine
* Tomatoes
* Watermelon (seasonal)

Pantry

My pantry isn't very big, so I bought an extra shelf unit at an organizer store and set it in an empty corner near my kitchen. Our home might seem unconventional to most, with the aforementioned shelf unit and extra freezer (oh, and did I mention I have two refrigerators?), but I don't care. I think it's awesome.

* Agave nectar
* Assortment of herbal teas
* Coconut oil
* Dried mushrooms
* Himalayan crystal salt
* Homemade sun-dried-tomato powder
* Olive oil
* Raw coconut crystals and raw coconut nectar

* Raw granola, kale chips, crackers, and snack bars
* Seeds for sprouting (alfalfa, mung, broccoli, and red clover)
* Stevia
* Sun-dried tomatoes
* Vanilla powder and flavoring extracts (almond, cherry, peppermint, coconut, maple, orange, lemon, etc.)
* Yacón syrup

Spices

I have around thirty assorted spices and herbs in my kitchen cabinet, but the must-haves are:

* Black pepper
* Cayenne pepper
* Cinnamon
* Cumin
* Curry powder
* Dill (dried)
* Garlic powder
* Ginger (ground)
* Italian seasoning
* Mexican seasoning and/or chili powder
* Nutmeg
* Onion powder

A Note About Herbs

Hands down, fresh herbs taste better and have higher nutritional value than dried herbs. (If possible, grow them yourself!) While I recommend fresh herbs whenever possible, you can substitute dried herbs if necessary. Do so in a ratio of 3 parts fresh to 1 part dried. Dried herbs impart a more concentrated flavor, which is why you need less of them. For instance, if your recipe calls for 3 tablespoons of minced fresh basil, use 1 tablespoon of dried basil instead.

RIPENESS, STORAGE, AND OTHER TIPS FOR FRESH PRODUCE

To truly experience the greatest health, it's important to eat fruits and vegetables at their peak of ripeness. I use Evert Fresh Green bags (available in your produce aisle or online) to store certain foods in my refrigerator, such as bell peppers, cucumbers, celery, carrots, apples, cabbage, lettuce (if it's not prebagged), and more.

APPLES

These should be firm to hard. Cold temperatures keep apples from continuing to ripen after they are picked, so you can keep them on your counter for a few days and then move them to the refrigerator. If possible, buy locally grown organic apples as close to harvesting as possible. Most apples that have traveled a distance to get to you have been in storage for months in your grocer's refrigerator. You can taste the difference.

AVOCADOS

Keep avocados on the counter until they ripen. To achieve quicker ripening, they can be placed in a loosely closed paper bag. When ripe, their skin is usually dark in color and if you gently squeeze one, it should give just a little. Once they're ripe, place them in the refrigerator, where they'll last up to a week longer. If you just keep them on the counter, they'll usually only last another couple of days. Ripening avocados give off a gas that could affect the ripening process of your other produce, so you might want to keep them separately. And, as with bananas, if you have a lot of avocados, you should split them up. This will help prevent all of your avocados from ripening at the same time.

BANANAS

If you're like most people, you probably think that a banana should be eaten when it is yellow. Nope. A truly ripe banana is one that has brown freckles or spots on the peel. This is the best, most flavorful, and healthiest time to eat a banana. Once you become accustomed to how ripe bananas are supposed to taste, you'll notice that yellow bananas seem starchy, less sweet, less flavorful, and almost coat the roof of your mouth with a waxy paste. This is because they aren't quite ripe, which also makes them harder to digest.

Store your bananas on your countertop away from other produce, because bananas, like avocados, give off a gas (ethylene) as they ripen, which can hasten the ripening process of your other produce. If you have a lot of bananas, split them up. This will help prevent all of your bananas from ripening at once. A ripe banana can be stored in the refrigerator for up to 4 days, but don't be surprised if the peel turns dark—this doesn't harm the banana. Another great tip for ripe bananas is to freeze them. All you have to do is peel the banana and freeze it in a baggie, pushing out as much air as possible (for best results, I always use a FoodSaver). When you are ready to use the banana, take it out and let it thaw for a few minutes. Frozen bananas are best used in raw ice creams or smoothies. Freezing them allows you to buy in bulk when prices are good.

BELL PEPPERS

I eat tons of red, orange, and yellow bell peppers, but not green varieties. Not only can their lack of ripeness be masked by their green color, but they are also less nutritious. For instance, red bell peppers have twice the vitamin C of green peppers and nine times the level of carotene and lycopene. Make sure your red, orange, or yellow bell peppers are fully ripe (no green areas), and store them in the refrigerator.

BERRIES

Do not wash berries until you are ready to eat them. They should always be stored in the refrigerator. Blueberries can last up to a week, but other berries should usually be eaten within a few days of purchase.

CITRUS

Lemons and oranges can be stored at room temperature for up to 1 week without refrigeration (or up to 3 weeks in the refrigerator). Limes should be refrigerated because they are more perishable.

DATES

Fresh dates should be somewhat smooth-skinned, glossy, plump, and soft; they should not be deeply wrinkled, leathery, broken, or cracked. They can be stored in the refrigerator in mason jars to prevent them from absorbing odors from other foods. They will last for up to 8 months.

FIGS

Good figs are plump and unbruised, with a mild fragrance and unbroken skin. Ripe fresh figs can be kept in the refrigerator for up to a week, or for a few days on the countertop.

FUYU PERSIMMONS

Look for deeply colored fruits, which should be more reddish than yellow. Buy glossy, well-rounded persimmons that are free of cracks or bruises, with their leaf-like sepals still green and attached. Ripe persimmons should be stored in the refrigerator and used as soon as possible.

KIWI

Did you know you can eat the whole fruit with the skin? Personally, I peel the skin off kiwis because I can't deal with the furriness, but some people eat the whole thing, skin and all. The best kiwis are plump, fragrant, and yield to gentle pressure. Unripe kiwis have a hard core and a very tart taste. To ripen kiwis, let them sit at room temperature for a few days.

MANGOES

The skin of mangoes can be toxic for some people, because this fruit belongs to the poison ivy family. You can tell if you are sensitive to mangoes by simply touching the skin and seeing if you get a rash or any skin irritation. Even if you do get a rash, most people who are sensitive to the skin of a mango can still eat the flesh inside with no problem. I usually keep mangoes on my counter for a few days to ripen, if needed. When they start to turn red and yellow in spots and they "give" a little when pressed, I move them to the refrigerator. A ripe mango will have a nice, intense fragrance.

PEARS

These should look relatively unblemished, with a nice, full color. In some varieties, full color will not develop until the fruit ripens. Pears are picked unripe and are usually hard. They can be stored at room temperature first to ripen, then refrigerated for no longer than a day or two before eating them. Ripe pears will give slightly to gentle pressure.

PINEAPPLE

A pineapple is ripe and ready for eating when you can no longer lift it by one of its leaves without the leaf coming off. It should also have a sweet smell. (Color is not always the best indicator, except that the leaves shouldn't be brown or dried). Test your pineapple for ripeness at the store to help ensure you're buying a sweet one. Just start pulling on the leaves. After three or four attempts on different leaves, if you can't gently take one of them out, move on to another pineapple.

STONE FRUITS (PEACHES, PLUMS, NECTARINES, APRICOTS, AND SO ON)

When ripe, these will "give" a little when gently pressed, but without a mushy feel. If they are hard, they aren't ripe. Ripen by leaving them on your counter at room temperature.

TOMATOES

Buy tomatoes that feel heavy for their size and are uniform in color. Fully ripe tomatoes should yield to gentle pressure. These are best stored on your countertop. Tomatoes give off the same gas (ethylene) as bananas and avocados. Do not put them in the refrigerator or they will develop a mealy texture. To make them last as long as possible, I store mine between two paper towels on a glass plate.

FREEZING PRODUCE

When you freeze your own fresh fruit and veggies, you can lose up to 30 percent of the nutritional value. However, that's not so bad when you look at the bigger picture. Even sitting on the counter, fresh fruit and veggies lose some of their nutrients. Eating frozen produce is much better than eating cooked food, which has lost the vast majority of its nutritional value. So, if you need to freeze some foods because you were able to buy them on sale and save money, then by all means do it! This is the kind of thing that helps you succeed with raw because it ensures you have lots of ingredients on hand, making it easier for you to prepare dishes whenever you want. Again, having a separate freezer makes this more feasible, especially when it comes to loading up on something when you find a great price.

The nutritional pros and cons of frozen *fruit* (not vegetables) are somewhat disputed. While some sources say frozen fruit has less nutritional value, others say it has more because the fruit was picked and frozen at its optimal ripeness and hasn't degraded from being shipped and sitting out on the supermarket shelves waiting to be purchased.

The same does *not* apply for commercially frozen vegetables. When you buy frozen vegetables, such as corn or peas, you always get less nutritional value. This is because frozen vegetables are blanched prior to freezing, which destroys most of the enzymes and nutrients.

DRIED HERBS

Dehydrating herbs is easy and rewarding. All you have to do is wash fresh herbs, dry them with a paper towel, and dehydrate them until thoroughly dry. If you're using an Excalibur dehydrator, it is helpful to place a mesh screen on top of the herbs while drying. When they are almost completely dry, they'll be light in weight, and the mesh screen ensures they won't fly around inside the dehydrator as the air blows. Store the whole dried leaves in a mason jar for up to 6 months and take them out as needed. When you are ready to use them, crush the leaves with your fingers, or use a mortar and pestle. Do not crush more than you need; it's best to store dehydrated herbs in the whole-leaf form to maintain the fullest flavor.

FRESH HERBS

The drier the leaves, the longer fresh herbs will keep, so don't wash them before you store them. The best storage method is in a plastic bag or packed loosely in a mason jar in your refrigerator's crisper. If the herbs are just harvested, most of them should remain in good shape for well over a week. Herbs with tough leaves like rosemary, thyme, and sage can keep for 2 weeks or more.

LEAFY GREENS

My favorite way to store leafy greens is to tear them into bite-size pieces (or cut the leaves using my ceramic knife because it doesn't cause oxidation where the knife cuts) and give them a good wash in cold water. Then, I use my salad spinner to dry the leafy greens and store the salad spinner, with the leafy greens inside, in my refrigerator. If I have more leafy greens than room in my salad spinner, I wash and dry them, wrap them in a paper towel, and store them in plastic bags.

Chard, micro greens, and bok choy should be stored in plastic bags in the refrigerator without being washed first.

SWEETENERS

The healthiest sweeteners are fresh fruits, such as berries, banana, mango, papaya, peaches, figs, dates, and so on. In addition to sweetness, they offer great nutritional value. But, of course, fresh fruit is not right for every recipe calling for some sweetness.

To sweeten recipes that aren't meant to be "fruity" or overly wet, raw fooders never use sugar, not even so-called "raw" sugar (which in this case means unrefined rather than unheated). Instead, we usually turn to one of two favorites: pitted fresh dates or raw agave nectar. Each of these has its advantages and disadvantages, so the best choice depends on how you're planning to use it.

Dates vs. Agave Nectar

Dates are a fruit, but they pack so much concentrated sweetness that I like to call them "nature's candy." A whole food that's loaded with calcium and magnesium, fresh dates are considered to be healthier than raw agave nectar. I love the organic Medjool dates from BlueMountainOrganics.com, and I buy them in a 5-pound (2.3-kg) bag. They are big, plump, and soft. But dates are a dense, chunky ingredient that can compromise the texture of some dishes.

Raw agave nectar is the juice of the agave plant (one variety of which is used to make tequila) that has been reduced to a syrup that's sweeter than honey but less viscous. (There is some debate among raw fooders as to whether raw agave nectar is truly raw, even when the label says "raw." To be safe, make sure the label also says it has not been heated over 118°F

[48°C]. For links to my favorite brands, visit KristensRaw.com/store.)

Raw agave nectar is very sweet and easy to work with because it's a liquid, meaning it stores easily in a bottle and mixes well in recipes. That said, it's not as nutritious as dates.

As a chef, I want great texture in my dishes and sometimes avoid using dates as a sweetener if I'm looking for absolute smoothness. But as a healthy-food advocate, I actually prefer fresh dates, even if they might add a little unwanted chunkiness to an otherwise smooth mixture.

As somebody who helps people embrace a raw vegan lifestyle, I'm supportive of helping them transition gradually, in baby steps, if necessary, and making it as easy as possible. You could say the "baby step" of sweeteners in raw food cuisine is raw agave nectar. Even though it's not as healthful as dates, it's easier to use and still healthier than most sweeteners used in the Standard American Diet, such as sugar or high-fructose corn syrup.

For convenience, you'll see that some of my recipes call for raw agave nectar. However, in most cases (especially where smooth texture is less important), you can substitute pitted dates in place of the agave nectar, especially if you're looking for optimal nutrition. Simply substitute 1 to 2 pitted dates for each tablespoon of raw agave nectar. Or if a recipe calls for ½ cup (120 ml) of raw agave, you can substitute 8 to 10 pitted dates (or more).

Dates won't give you a super-creamy texture, but the texture can be improved by including an intermediate step: making a "date paste" (see recipe, below). This takes a little extra time, and of course, you need to have dates on hand—yet another reason many raw fooders just reach for the bottle of agave nectar instead.

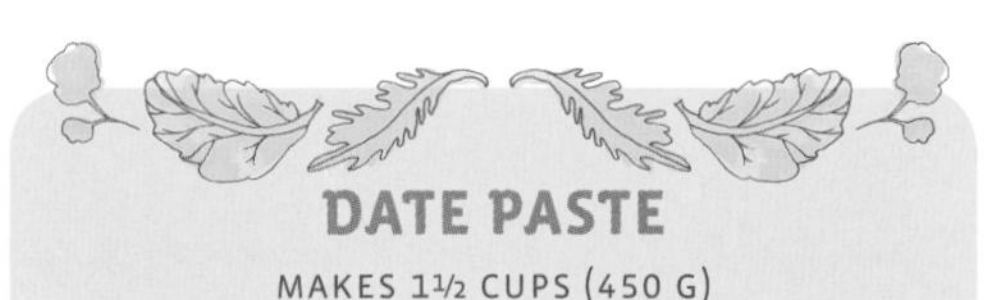

DATE PASTE

MAKES 1½ CUPS (450 G)

It's great to keep this on hand in the refrigerator. Date paste is easy to make and takes less than 10 minutes to prepare once the dates are soaked.

15 MEDJOOL DATES, PITTED
2 CUPS (480 ML) WATER (FOR SOAKING)

Put the dates in a bowl and add the water. Let soak for 30 minutes. Drain, reserving the soaking water. Add the dates and ½ cup (120 ml) of the reserved soaking water to a food processor and puree to a smooth paste. Store it in an airtight container in the refrigerator for up to 10 days.

Other Raw Sweeteners

The following is a list of sweeteners that can be used in my recipes in place of dates and raw agave nectar.

HONEY

Most honey found in conventional supermarkets is heated, but most found in natural foods stores is technically raw (consult the label when in doubt). However, honey is not considered vegan because it is produced by bees and is therefore an animal by-product. While honey does not have the health risks associated with animal by-products such as eggs or dairy, it can spike the body's natural sugar levels. Both agave nectar and coconut nectar have a healthier glycemic index and can be substituted for honey in any recipe in a 1-to-1 ratio.

MAPLE SYRUP

Maple syrup is made from the boiled sap of the maple tree. It is not considered raw, but some people still use it as a sweetener.

RAW CHOCOLATE

I love the fact that one of my greatest pleasures in life—chocolate—is actually good for me, in moderation, of course. Raw chocolate is made from cacao beans and is unrefined, unprocessed, all natural, and filled with nutrients. I always buy Navitas Naturals raw chocolate powder and cacao nibs.

RAW COCONUT CRYSTALS

Also called coconut sugar, this interesting sweetener is subtly sweet and has a low glycemic rating (35) and a good nutrient profile. It contains seventeen amino acids, broad-spectrum B vitamins, and more. Coconut crystals are great to use in raw cobblers and shakes. I buy the Coconut Secret brand at Whole Foods Market.

RAW COCONUT NECTAR

Also called coconut syrup, this sweetener, much like raw coconut crystals, has a low glycemic index of 35 and contains the same nutrients. Use it in shakes, smoothies, desserts, teas, and more. Usually you can interchange this sweetener with raw agave nectar in recipes.

RAW VANILLA POWDER

One of my favorite ingredients is raw vanilla powder. I find myself adding it to almost all of my smoothies, shakes, and desserts. If you're a fan of vanilla, you must stock this in your kitchen. It's available at most Whole Foods Markets, but you can get a better price on Amazon.com. See my store for details: KristensRaw.com/store.

STEVIA

This sugar substitute is made from the leaf of the stevia plant. It has a sweet taste but is low in calories and doesn't elevate blood sugar levels. It's very sweet, so you'll want to use much less stevia than you would any other sweetener. My mom actually grows her own stevia. It's a way to add sweetness to dishes like fresh smoothies without adding calories. If you can't grow your own, I recommend Navitas Naturals' organic stevia. It's the best-tasting stevia I've found.

YACÓN SYRUP

This sweetener has a low glycemic index and a nice molasses-type flavor. You can replace raw agave nectar with this sweetener, but note that raw agave nectar is sweeter. My favorite brand is Navitas Naturals, available at NavitasNaturals.com.

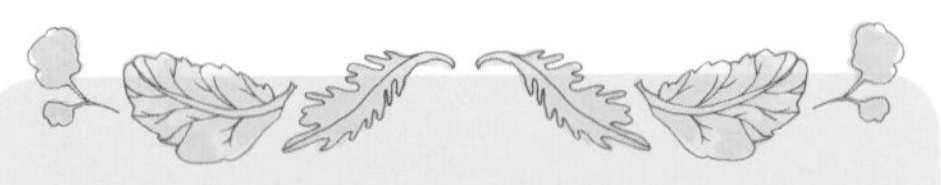

LIQUID MEASUREMENTS

1 tablespoon = 3 teaspoons
1 ounce (30 ml) = 2 tablespoons
¼ cup (60 ml/2 fl oz) = 4 tablespoons
⅓ cup (80 ml/2½ fl oz) = 5⅓ tablespoons
½ cup (120 ml/4 fl oz) = 8 tablespoons
1 cup (240 ml/8 fl oz) = 16 tablespoons or ½ pint
2 cups (480 ml/16 fl oz) = 1 pint
4 cups (960 ml/32 fl oz) = 1 quart
16 cups (3.8 l) = 4 quarts or 1 gallon

SOAKING AND DEHYDRATING RAW FOODS

Nuts and Seeds

When using nuts and seeds in raw vegan foods, you'll find that recipes sometimes call for them to be soaked or soaked and dehydrated. Here is the low-down on the difference between the two techniques.

Why Should You Soak Your Nuts and Seeds?

Most nuts and seeds come packed by Mother Nature with enzyme inhibitors, rendering them harder to digest. These inhibitors essentially shut down the nuts' and seeds' metabolic activity, rendering them dormant—for as long as they need to be—until they detect a moisture-rich environment that's suitable for germination (such as moist soil).

By soaking your nuts and seeds, you trick the nuts into "waking up," thus shutting off the inhibitors so that the enzymes can become active. This greatly enhances the nuts' digestibility and is highly recommended if you want to experience raw vegan food in the healthiest way possible.

Even though you'll want to soak the nuts to activate their enzymes, before using them you might need to re-dry them and grind them anywhere from coarse to fine (into a powder almost like flour), depending on the recipe. To dry them, you'll need a dehydrator (instructions follow). However, if you don't yet own a dehydrator, just skip the soaking part of a recipe calling for soaking and dehydrating. You can use the nuts or seeds in the dry form that you bought them.

Soaking and dehydrating nuts is ideal before storing them in the freezer or refrigerator. They will last a long time and you'll always have them on hand, ready to use, in the most digestible fashion. You can then grind them to the consistency called for in the recipe.

Some nuts and seeds don't have enzyme inhibitors (macadamia nuts, Brazil nuts, pine nuts, hemp seeds, and most cashews) and therefore generally don't need to be soaked, but you still might want to if you're trying to make them easier to blend. (This is helpful when making nut milks, dressings, soups, and sauces. Exception: Hemp seeds and pine nuts are quite soft without soaking, so you can usually just use these as is.)

Flaxseeds and Chia Seeds

Flaxseeds and chia seeds don't need to be soaked if your recipe calls for grinding them into a powder. Some recipes will call for soaking the seeds in their "whole-seed" form before making crackers and bread, because they create a very gelatinous and binding texture when soaked. You can soak these seeds in a ratio of 1 part seeds to 2 parts water, and they can be soaked for as little as 1 hour and as much as up to 12 hours. At this point, they are ready to use (don't drain them). Personally, when I use flaxseeds, I usually grind them and don't soak them. It's hard for your body to digest "whole" flaxseeds, even if they are soaked. It's easier for your body to assimilate the nutrients when they're ground to a flax meal.

Instructions for Soaking Nuts and Seeds

When a recipe in this book calls for 1 cup (115 g) of seeds or nuts, do the following:

Put 1 cup (115 g) seeds or nuts in a bowl. Add water to cover by 1 inch (2.5 cm). Let stand at room temperature for the time designated in the recipe. Drain and rinse the seeds or nuts, discarding the soaking water, which will contain enzyme inhibitors.

The seeds or nuts are now ready to use in the recipe. If you can't make the recipe immediately, you can keep the seeds or nuts in a covered container in the refrigerator for up to three days. To prevent them from drying out, give them a daily rinse.

When a recipe requires soaking, here are the average times for various nuts and seeds:

* Almonds: 12 hours
* Cashews, Brazil nuts, macadamia nuts, and pine nuts: 1 to 2 hours
* Sunflower seeds and pumpkin seeds: 6 to 8 hours
* Walnuts and pecans: 6 to 8 hours

Dehydrating Nuts

After soaking, draining, and rinsing nuts, spread them out on a mesh dehydrator sheet and dehydrate them at 130° to 140°F (54° to 60°C) for about 1 hour. Then, reduce the temperature to 105° to 110°F (40° to 43°C), and continue dehydrating them until they're completely dry, which can take up to 24 hours.

Soaking and Sprouting Buckwheat Groats

Buckwheat groats double in volume after they've been soaked (before dehydrating). For example, if a recipe calls for 2 cups (320 g) buckwheat groats (soaked), then it means that you will start with about 1 cup (85 g) dry buckwheat groats.

To soak and sprout buckwheat groats: Put 1 cup (85 g) dry buckwheat groats in a bowl. Add water to cover by 1 inch (2.5 cm). Let soak at room temperature for 8 to 12 hours. Drain, rinse well, and transfer to a colander set over a bowl (to catch the dripping water). Gently cover the colander with a paper towel and let the buckwheat sprout for 24 to 36 hours, rinsing it about every 12 hours. Makes 2 cups (320 g) sprouted buckwheat.

If you have leftover sprouted buckwheat, simply place it on a dehydrator tray and dehydrate until dry (about 24 hours). Eat plain, in trail mix, as a raw cereal, stirred into vegan yogurt, or sprinkled over salad. Crunchy delightfulness!

Soaking Dried Fruits

Some recipes call for rehydrated dried fruits such as goji berries, golden berries, prunes, and raisins. To rehydrate dried fruits, put them in a bowl and add water to cover by about ½ inch (12 mm). Let soak at room temperature for 30 to 60 minutes, or until soft. Reserve the soaking water to drink or to use later in the recipe.

Sun-Dried Tomatoes

By far the best "sun"-dried tomatoes are those you make yourself in a dehydrator. If you don't have a dehydrator, make sure you buy "dry-pack" sun-dried tomatoes, usually found in the bulk section of your natural foods market. Don't buy the sun-dried tomatoes that are packed in a jar of oil. Also, don't buy sun-dried tomatoes if they're really dark (almost black), because these don't taste as good.

Again, I recommend making sun-dried tomatoes yourself if you truly want the freshest flavor possible. It's really fun to do! And it's super easy. Plus, it saves money. Simply slice organic tomatoes and dehydrate them in your dehydrator until dry. The thinner you slice them, the faster they will dry.

Soaking Sun-Dried Tomatoes

To soak sun-dried tomatoes, put them in a bowl and add water to cover by ½ to ¾ inch (12 mm to 2 cm). Let soak at room temperature for 15 to 60 minutes or until soft; the time will vary, depending on the thickness of the slices. Drink the soaking water, or reserve it for later use in the recipe.

Because I make my sun-dried tomatoes thin, I can break them with my hands, which is what I do before soaking them in some recipes. If you use store-bought sun-dried tomatoes, they will probably be thicker and harder to break (or cut) before soaking. Therefore, I recommend soaking them first, and then chopping them after they're done soaking, if needed.

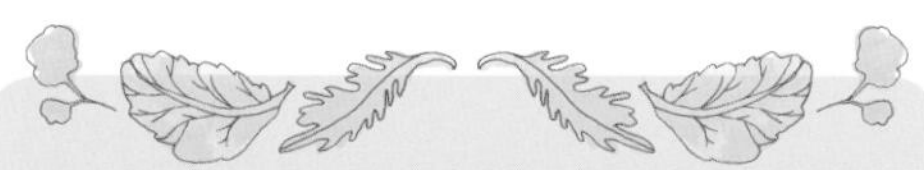

WHAT IS THE DIFFERENCE BETWEEN CHOPPED, DICED, AND MINCED?

Chop: To cut a food into relatively uniform cuts that are not perfectly neat or even. You'll often be asked to chop something before putting it into a blender or food processor; it doesn't have to be uniform size since it will be blended or pureed.

Dice: To cut a food into an even cube shape of different sizes. Used for foods that will be served with their diced shape intact.

Mince: To very finely chop a food such as fresh herbs, garlic, and fresh ginger.

Julienne: To cut a food into matchstick shapes.

MASON JARS

I store as much food as I can in mason jars. They are better for the environment and a healthier alternative to plastic, much of which has chemicals that can seep into food. Mason jars are inexpensive and can be found at most hardware stores, grocery stores, and online. I store nuts, seeds, and unsweetened coconut in mason jars in the freezer. My raw breads and crackers are stored in the freezer, too, if I don't plan on eating them within two weeks of making them. I store dates, raisins, and other dried fruits in mason jars as well. It's a smart idea to label everything with the contents and the date—trust me, you *will* forget. You can write on mason jars with a Sharpie permanent marker. Don't worry, it's not actually permanent; it scrubs off easily with a little dish soap and a sponge. To really get into the habit of regularly storing things, I recommend buying a few dozen mason jars. You'll want a range of sizes. One-cup, quart, and half-gallon (250-ml, 1-l, and 2-l) wide-mouth mason jars are the best.

START SPROUTING!

"Sprouting" means to cultivate seeds in a non-soil environment just long enough for them to "wake up" from their dormant stage, burst into life, and sprout tiny stems and leaves—and then you eat them! It's also a perfect way to keep yourself on the raw food path.

I'm going to let you in on a little secret (the gardeners among you might know this already): aside from the physical/health benefits of eating sprouts (which many people speak about), one of the best things about sprouting is what it does for your *mental* outlook. The process of growing your own sprouts is amazing! When I walk into my kitchen every day and see these little greenish babies growing from seeds to fresh sprouts, it makes me smile and I'm reminded of the pure, "living" lifestyle I lead. It's impossible to forget, because these little foods are growing before my eyes, literally changing daily. Seeing sprouts grow inspires me and imbues me with a kind of energy, like a ray of light, that is hard to describe but is every bit as real as the nutritional benefits of these foods.

And sprouts are super-nutritious. Add them to salads, smoothies, and soups; eat them plain; top your pâté with them; take them in a baggie in your car—basically, eat them every chance you get!

Sprouting is fairly simple. It involves soaking seeds overnight, draining, and placing them in jars turned upside-down, tilted at an angle to let moisture drip out of special mesh lids. Rinse the sprouts once or twice a day for several days, until the sprouts have grown to the length you prefer. To see how it's done, check out my video at: KristensRaw.com/sprouts.

CHAPTER 10

DEALING WITH CRAVINGS

The more you know, and the more you learn over time, the more confident and empowered you will feel about choosing to live the raw lifestyle. We are bombarded with advertising every minute of the day for processed, cooked, unhealthful, and addictive foods. We need this armor of raw food knowledge to shield ourselves and stand tall, saying "no" to unhealthy cravings and foods.

The pain of discipline is much easier than the pain of regret.
—Jim Rohn

DON'T WORRY—IT'S NOT GOING ANYWHERE

Here is a great trick: Remember that if you are craving a certain food, "it's not going anywhere." It wasn't that long ago that our ancestors were barely scraping out a living, just trying to find enough food to survive. Before agriculture, food availability was irregular, and our bodies were well adapted to this, with the ability to convert extra food into fat that would carry us through lean times, such as every winter. That feature of our physiology was good back then and helped us to survive. Unfortunately, in a world with abundant food, it works against us, and in fact is killing us by the millions. Our natural instincts tell us to eat, eat, eat, even when we're not hungry, in order to store calories in our bodies. But our society has managed to eliminate those times of scarcity. This is a recipe for obesity!

Among other things, cravings are the body's way of telling you to store food "in case you run out." (And the effect is even worse for people who grew up in a large family!)

Fortunately, you have the power to use your thinking brain to override your instincts. One of the best things you can tell yourself the next time you're experiencing a craving is that "the food isn't going anywhere." It will always be there later if you want it. This simple little mental trick will enable you to step back and take a look at the bigger picture. This really works, even if you have to say the words out loud: "I can always have this later if I want."

Here is an exercise that is very effective: The next time you want to give in to a craving for something unhealthful, take a moment to reflect on the following, even if it's while you're in line to buy whatever it is you "think" you need at that moment:

Do I really want this? Maybe I do. But, should I have it? If so, why? Do I have to have it now? How would I feel if I came back later tonight or even tomorrow? Would I still want it? If so, why don't I try that? I realize that it is not going anywhere (Taco Bell, Starbucks, popcorn at the movies, whatever it is), *and I can have it at a later date. I'll just say "no" for now.*

I was amazed at how many times I was comfortable with saying "no" to myself in that moment because I knew I could have the food later, *if* I even wanted it later. I left myself that option, which eliminated the feeling of deprivation. This made me comfortable, and it worked. What's even better is that it was a very rare occasion that I went back for it at a later time. I was empowered by having said "no" to an addiction.

It always helps to make the object of your craving inconvenient to access. The more times you do this, the stronger your mind gets, and the less addicted you are because you're not putting substances in your body that you'll end up having to deal with at a later date. Success begets success, and eventually, discipline isn't required because you will have developed a habit of not eating bad food.

BEING PREPARED

There might be times when you're craving a certain food. When those times come, be prepared. Studies show that cravings are often fleeting and go as quickly as they come. In fact, they often pass in as little as five minutes. One way to ensure this is to immediately distract yourself by doing something else—anything.

Jumping rope for a couple of minutes is great, or playing with an app on your iPhone. I love reading books on my iPhone with the Kindle app, and I have plenty of motivating healthy-eating books on it. If I feel a craving coming on, I get out my phone and start looking at some highlighted passages to motivate me. Craving passes. Disaster averted. I like thinking about a quote from Frank Herbert's *Dune* during these times, but I replace the word *fear* with *craving*:

I will face my fear (craving). *I will permit it to pass over me and through me. And when it has gone past I will turn the inner eye to see its path. Where the fear* (craving) *has gone there will be nothing. Only I will remain.*

CRAVING REPLACEMENT OPTIONS

Here is a list of foods to try so you do not indulge in the actual craving. If you crave the item on the left, then replace it with the raw vegan food(s) on the right:

TYPICAL CRAVING	RAW REPLACEMENT
CAFFEINE, DRUGS, ALCOHOL	"Plant Blood," a.k.a. fresh green juice, fresh carrot juice, fresh apple juice, fresh orange juice
CARAMEL	Raw carob, dates, or dried Turkish figs
CHEESE	Raw nut/seed cheese or cheese spread
CHIPS AND DIP	Raw hummus, ranch dip, dehydrated zucchini chips
CHOCOLATE	Raw chocolate
DESSERT	Dates stuffed with nuts, or any raw dessert
FISH AND SUSHI	Nori rolls, sea vegetables
ICE CREAM	Raw ice cream
ITALIAN FOOD	Raw pasta or lasagna
JELL-O OR FRUIT-FLAVORED CANDY	Fruit smoothie, fruit, dates

MEAT, RICE, BEANS	Raw nut pâté, raw hummus with veggies, flax bread with raw cheese spread, raw marinated mushrooms
MEXICAN FOOD	Nut pâté with Mexican seasoning
MILK	Raw nut/seed milk
MILKSHAKE	Raw nut/seed milk with crushed ice or frozen banana
PASTRY	Raw granola
PIZZA	Raw pizza
PROTEIN SHAKE SUPPLEMENT	Raw hemp milk or raw protein shake (see below)
SUGAR	Fruit smoothie

PROTEIN POWDERS: A POWERFUL WEAPON AGAINST CRAVINGS

Not too long ago, there weren't a lot of protein powder options for raw vegans. Fortunately, due to the skyrocketing popularity of raw food, there's been a lot of innovation in recent years, and I'm happy to report that raw fooders now have several great options when it comes to protein powder. They run the gamut from brown rice protein and Brazil nut protein to hemp protein and all kinds of mixtures with ideal ratios of all eight essential amino acids. (This area is evolving constantly, so for up-to-date recommendations of brands of protein powder, visit KristensRaw.com/store.)

I know what a lot of you are thinking: "Protein powder? Yuck." Protein powders get mixed reviews from people. Some people don't care for protein powders because they're a "fractionated food" (not a whole food). There are other people, however, like me, who are grateful they exist. Some raw folks love them because they want more protein in their diets to support their intense exercise regime (such as my husband, or Robert Cheeke, a vegan bodybuilder). Other people, like me, love them when pregnant or breastfeeding for that easy extra protein. But that's not the only reason I like them.

When I'm eating an all-raw diet (breastfeeding, pregnant, or not), I find there are times I want a food that is neither high carbohydrate nor high fat. A lot of raw foods are either one of those two options. Sure, I could gnaw on some plain romaine or cucumbers, but that's not going to fill me up or satisfy the need for something substantial and filling but not high fat (there go nuts) or high carb (sorry, fruit). I've heard the same thing from many of my readers. So, how do I handle it? I drink a protein shake. And it's exactly what I need!

Now, I realize that some people just have a hard time getting into protein drinks, even if they are interested in the idea, because of the chalky texture or the flavor. But I'm accustomed to the texture (of course, I've been drinking protein shakes for some twenty years now, because they were a big part of my bodybuilding regimen). I'm used to them and have been for a long time. But then something more profound happened: now I even crave the stuff sometimes. I know, weird, right? Craving a plain protein shake? Just the powder and water shaken up? Yes! The secret: Once I consciously realized that this drink indeed filled a physical need for me, it mentally satisfied me. It also filled me up, which is great for anyone watching calories. It was the perfect solution to keeping my diet raw without eating more carbs or fat when that wasn't what my body was asking for.

All of the above comes much more easily, of course, if you start by finding a protein powder that you like (my husband loves chocolate-flavored varieties). If you're one of those people who can't imagine drinking plain protein powder mixed with water, try some of the following suggestions to see if they help:

* **Blend the powder with water and ice or really cold water.** I find that when the shake is really cold, I enjoy it more. If the water from your tap isn't cold enough and you don't want to use ice, either keep a pitcher of cold water in your refrigerator or make the shake in advance and chill it before drinking.

* **Add pizzazz.** I love adding ¼ to ½ teaspoon of ground cinnamon to my protein powder shakes. Sometimes I add nutmeg, too. Raw vanilla powder is fun, as are other flavors like almond, orange, or peppermint extract. Add cayenne and give your circulation a boost! Get creative and diversify the flavors so they're not always the same. You can even get extra wild and add garam masala or fenugreek or curry powder.

* **Add extra water.** At the time of this writing, my whole family drinks Sun Warrior's Chocolate protein powder. My mom likes hers with more water, and she enjoys each sip of it as she takes her time drinking it. I tend to make mine thicker and drink it faster. My husband chugs his whole shake down in a series of gulps without coming up for air three to four times a day.

* **Mix it with raw coconut water or raw almond milk for variety.**

Before I realized that protein shakes were a perfect solution, I used to sit there and think, "I'm hungry. No, I don't want a bunch of nuts.

No, I don't feel like sugar from fruits. No, I need something more than a huge bowl of plain romaine. I think cooked black beans or lentils would do the trick but I want to keep it raw right now. Hmmm . . ." That's when I decided to drink a protein shake one night because I was out of options. Well, it worked. I was full and satisfied. I was excited because it was a way for me to stick to the raw diet and be happy without filling up on foods I wasn't in the mood for.

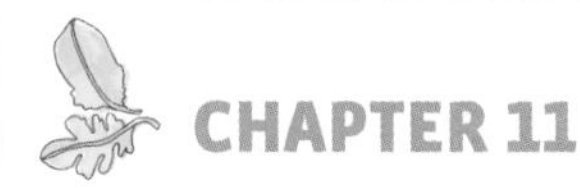

CHAPTER 11

SETTING YOURSELF UP TO SUCCEED WITH THE RAW FOOD LIFESTYLE

With a little bit of knowledge, going raw is a lot of fun. I mean, think about it: learning how to *not cook* food is a lot easier than learning how to cook food!

That said, some people have a hard time snapping out of their old habits. Often, the path of least resistance is what is most familiar. Also, people around you can either be a source of encouragement or a source of friction, depending on their attitude about striving for optimal health or trying new things in general (you know who I'm talking about—there's at least one in every family). This chapter is all about tips and tricks that have helped me and my clients succeed with the raw food lifestyle.

KNOW YOUR OUTCOME AND MEASURE YOUR PROGRESS

In any endeavor in life, knowing your outcome ahead of time is one of the most important things you can do for yourself.

So let's begin by envisioning what you want to look and feel like. Set a goal. Close your eyes for a moment and just think about this. Feel it. Pretend you have a magic wand—what would you do with it? What kinds of things would you change about yourself, your health, your body, and your energy? Think about how you will feel when you are at your desired weight. Think about how you will look, the kind of clothes you will wear, and how they will fit your body. Think about how you will feel when you have an abundance of energy. Imagine feeling good inside and out, exuding vitality in every movement and action. Go on a walk and ponder why you're embarking on this raw food journey. Imagine yourself being pulled forward by a force outside yourself and getting lighter with every step. What is pulling you in this direction?

Remember these visions and thoughts. Keep them at the front of your mind. One way to do this is to spend part of your time in the shower thinking about these visions. It's the perfect setting: you're not distracted, and it's the first thing you do each day. Creating this mind-set at the start of each day is of fundamental importance.

Visions transform into goals when you commit them to paper. Write down your goals on sticky notes and stick them everywhere so they are always in your face, reminding you of the new "you" that you are becoming and the new "lifestyle" that you're living. Here are some examples to get you started:

* "Eat 100 percent raw for three days straight."
* "Do something physical every day."
* "Get up from my desk every hour and do 5 pushups."
* "Try 2 new raw recipes each week."

I placed these notes all over the place: refrigerator, car dashboard, computer, desk, bathroom mirror, nightstand—even in my purse and makeup bag. Then every time I looked at them I was reminded of my lifestyle and goals. It's empowering because it's always on your mind.

The next thing to do is to find something measurable and track it. A sense of progress is a key to motivation. You can track any number of things, from your blood analysis to weight on the scale and circumference of your waist to the strength of your bench press and distance run to the number of consecutive all-raw or high-raw days. Pick something, anything, big or small, and track it. This keeps you moving in the right direction.

Another great tip is to set modest goals that you can attain rather quickly. Save the big stuff until after you get your groove on and have built up momentum like a raw-food-chuggin' locomotive. Instead of setting the goal to eat a high-raw diet for life, set a goal to eat a high-raw diet two days a week. Instead of setting a goal to lose 20 pounds (9 kg), set a goal to lose 4 pounds (1.8 kg). Once you attain your goals, celebrate your awesome self! Then, set new goals. Setting goals in chunks like this makes them easier to attain, keeps the momentum going, and is a lot more fun.

BLOGGING: THE NEW JOURNALING

Keeping a daily journal that tracks what you eat, your exercise routine, and what you're thinking about with respect to these things is one of the best ways to stay on track. And, nowadays, the coolest way to do this is online with a blog.

Blogging is effective, for one main reason: feedback. Unlike a journal, when you blog, you tell the world. If you like, you can be anonymous by using a screen name or "handle" instead of your real name. Both real names and fictitious names are extremely common; it's a matter of personal preference (many people have one or more of each and talk about different things using different names, such as professional matters under their real name and politics or sports under a pseudonym like "sportsfan057").

When you tell the world, several important things happen: again, you get feedback. The most common form of feedback will be people leaving comments and questions on your blog. You can set it up so that the public either can or can't view the comments, or they can view them only after you've first approved the messages.

Also, you meet people—sometimes people will contact you directly via e-mail. (You can still maintain your anonymity if you like, by using a different e-mail address.) Because they're contacting you based on what you've written, their e-mails are frequently very relevant to the subject matter and what you're trying to do with raw. They may have questions they'd like to ask you, answers for questions that you've posed, suggestions you never would have thought of on your own, or they might just write to say "hi."

When you blog, you provide knowledge to others who may follow in your footsteps tomorrow or ten years from now. What you write might be archived and searchable for years—even decades—to come. In most endeavors in life, somebody else has already been there. Any problem you encounter, somebody else has already encountered—and solved. The collective wisdom of millions of people recording their experiences has immeasurable value to others.

But here is the *single most* important reason to maintain a blog: accountability. You're much more likely to stick with pursuing your goal. Perhaps a hundred times more likely, partly out of a sense of social obligation (keeping your promise to the world out there) and, again, because of feedback from that world—those are real people out there, after all. Studies show that people can lose 20 percent more weight, for instance, when announcing that commitment publicly, and a blog is the perfect way to do this. When you do it via a blog or online forum, your natural curiosity will start nagging at you, wondering whether anybody has left any comments. This curiosity alone reinforces the behavior. But when somebody actually writes something, especially something very reinforcing—look out! You'll be motivated to write more, leading to a positive feedback loop so profound in its impact on your behavior that you won't believe it.

To set up a blog, just go to blogspot.com and create a free account. It's easy and takes only five minutes. It doesn't have to be fancy; just get it up and start typing. Don't worry if you don't get feedback right away. Just keep writing. Eventually, people will find your blog, especially if it's about raw food, as there is quite an active raw food community online, and people are eager to search and reach out to one another. Start by going to other people's raw food blogs on blogspot.com and leaving comments, questions, and words of encouragement for them. This is a great way for people to find out about your blog (there will be a link to your blog when you post a message on their blog). Another great way to meet others with similar interests is by using Facebook and Twitter. Take it from me, when you post something minor but inspirational about what you're doing, and you come back a few hours later and see that a bunch of your Facebook friends have "liked" it, you'll feel a little endorphin drip of glowy satisfaction, making you want to keep on doing whatever it is you wrote about.

Keeping a blog about raw food and/or your life is one of the most rewarding things you can do. Once you start, you become addicted to it (in a good way). As you look back on it, you'll read it with pride, self-discovery, and fun. Over time, it will also become the chronicle and official record of your life. (What a gift to leave to your children, even if you don't have any yet!)

To start, keep track of every little success you have. You build on success, and this is how you reinforce your progress. Every time you look back and see progress, no matter how small, you'll be inspired to do more. Even if you are just starting out, you can write things like "I ate raw food for breakfast; I walked up and down my stairs two times," then later that day you write, "I ate mostly raw at lunch." This might sound simple, or too boring to blog about, but it's very important—it's tracking your progress and demonstrating to the world that people *actually do live this way*. When you look at it the following day, you'll know the next step you need to take to get to the next level.

Want to make it more adventurous and exciting? Make a bet! This can be done with people you know, and you can keep everyone updated with the details via your blog. For example, if you want to set a goal of losing 25 pounds (11.3 kg), bet your family, friends, and coworkers that you can do it in a set period of time. Chart your progress online. That's a sure way to stay on track.

TAKE PICTURES!

One of the best pieces of advice I can offer is to take tons of pictures. Take them all the time! Post them to your blog. The reason taking pictures works is right in line with setting yourself up to win and blogging. Take pictures of your countertop filled with fresh organic produce. It's okay to brag a little—it will inspire others. Have someone take pictures of you preparing raw food in your kitchen. Take pictures of yourself setting up a new appliance, and be sure to catch that beaming smile on your face—it will infect others with excitement! Take a picture to celebrate the cleaning out of your cupboards when you throw away the junk food. It's a great reminder so you don't buy that unhealthful food again. Take pictures of your body as you get healthier and healthier. Tape some of the pictures onto your kitchen cupboards, the fridge door, your bathroom mirror—even inside your car—for a reminder and motivation the next time you're buying produce or resisting a craving for whatever unhealthful food you happen to see.

SCHEDULE REWARDS IN ADVANCE

This one is fun: a reward list. Having a list of rewards that you can look forward to is another great way to set yourself up for victory. Write all the things you want and desire on a piece of paper. New kitchen equipment can be a great reward here, as it reinforces the raw lifestyle so powerfully. Even if you can't afford these things right now, still list them. Once you put something on paper, even if it is listed as a "reward" in your mind, it actually is a "goal," too. And as you probably know, a goal on paper starts to take on a life of its own, and you start moving toward that objective automatically—just by writing it down.

The next great tip is to schedule some of your rewards—in advance. This creates a sense of accountability. If you want a massage, and you need to earn it by being 100 percent raw for two weeks straight, then call the spa and schedule it. Write it on your calendar so you're constantly reminded of the reward.

Supporting and rewarding yourself for all wins, big and small, is crucial. This keeps you motivated. In the beginning, when I began my raw journey, I rewarded myself as much as possible. Every three days that I went 100 percent raw, I treated myself to new makeup or music or books and magazines (things that I love). Other ideas for rewards could be a kitchen appliance, a raw specialty food (truffle oil or raw chocolate), some new bath oils or soy candles. Even small, inexpensive items can make wonderfully satisfying rewards. After about four times of successfully sticking with 100 percent raw for three days, I was on a roll and I decided to up the ante by attempting to go raw for seven days straight, then two weeks, a month, and so on.

There also came a time when I knew I could—if I wanted to—make my reward a cooked vegan meal (this was a "mental reward" for me). Some purists might not agree with the philosophy behind it, but you have to do whatever works best for you, and this was something that worked for me—provided I didn't let it get out of control.

Cooked food can be addictive, so I had to set myself up to win if I did this. One of the ways I ensured this was to never buy any food in the store that requires cooking. After all, my microwave, stove, and oven were out of commission because they are used for storage anyway. And not keeping ingredients for cooked food in the house helps you avoid temptation. Keep in mind that this is generally important only during your transition to raw; there will come a time when you won't be tempted even if these foods are in your house.

It might seem counterintuitive to reward your physical efforts with something that doesn't seem to optimally support you physically, but here is where I'm a little different from many hard-core raw fooders. I'm aware that mental rewards are critical to success. I think scheduling a day (or meal) of food "treats" can be hugely motivating for staying on track all the other days.

However, this isn't the solution for everyone. I have clients who can't get off the raw path at all or they run the risk of falling off completely and losing control with cooked food. Or, maybe your goal is to always be 100 percent raw. If so, then you'll want to find other ways to reward yourself.

Maybe the best reward for you is to take some time for yourself to do the things you like to do. Maybe it's buying a magazine or treating yourself to an activity that you would not normally do, like spending a weekend at a resort or going on a hot air balloon ride. Or taking a day off work and going to a movie you've been dying to see. It doesn't matter what it is; just make sure you give yourself something to look forward to and set a date to do it by. If you feel like you are struggling during any point of the journey, all you have to do is look forward to the reward you're going to give yourself.

Some people might say, "Well, you shouldn't have to reward yourself. Your health should be the reward itself." Yes, this is fine and true for some—but, in the beginning stages, when this is all new to you and you find yourself too tired to make something raw and you just want to go through the Taco Bell drive-through, these little mental games can make all the difference in the world.

AVOIDING ROUTINE TEMPTATION

It will be much easier if you simply *avoid* foods that tempt you on a routine basis. The saying "Out of sight, out of mind" has never been truer than with unhealthful but tempting foods.

If you have to find a new route to work so you don't drive by your former favorite coffeehouse, then so be it. Or, if you have to avoid the movie theater because you are afraid you won't enjoy your movie without popcorn, then just avoid it for now. (Or, do what my mom does: she puts Vicks VapoRub under her nose so when she walks by the concession stand, she's not tempted by the smell of the popcorn—my mom has all kinds of crazy tricks like this.) Don't worry, such tactics are only temporary as you get used to your lifestyle. Avoiding temptations altogether helped accelerate my transition to raw food because I didn't think about things that tempted me nearly as much. I was able to stay focused on raw and its amazing health benefits. Feeling deprived was rarely an issue, because I no longer focused on the things I was no longer eating.

SOCIAL SITUATIONS AND PEER GROUPS

When it comes to the raw lifestyle, one of the biggest hurdles for people is social occasions. To this I say: *raise your standards*. This includes your peer group. Is this being ruthless? Not when you consider the consequences of the alternative: Premature death is ruthless. Real friends should support your decisions. People who don't aren't good friends, especially if they only see your decision to eat healthier as a judgment of how they choose to eat. The flip side of this is that you can't get preachy to them about their choices, although you certainly can try to lead by example or be there to answer questions. In my experience, there will always be a couple of people who think what you're doing is cool and want more information; a couple who think it's a good idea but not something they could do; a large group who are mostly indifferent; and a couple of people who get defensive about their own diet. That's just how the world is. This diverse range of reactions is normal, it's to be expected, and it's just no big deal if you don't let it be a big deal to you. And remember, you don't have to spend time around the naysayers if you don't want to.

Now, family is another issue. We don't get to choose who's in our family. Here are some nice words of wisdom: "Love your family and choose your peer group." That is, pick the latter wisely, not just befriending whoever happens to be around, as we tend to become like those we spend time with. This is one of the keys to setting yourself up to win. Your life is typically a reflection of your peer group's behaviors and expectations.

Whether family or friends, those around you might not be excited about what you are doing. The reason for this is because the changes you are making to better your health shine the light on *their* lifestyle choices. *Important:* This is not your problem, it's theirs. You might never say a word to them about their diet, but you will almost certainly encounter people who object to the idea of raw (and vegan in general) because they feel that *their* way of life is under scrutiny.

Food is a bizarrely emotionally loaded issue for many individuals. If you told people that you like, say, folk music, they wouldn't require that you defend your preference, or go on about how they must have their classic rock. However, if you told them that you only listened to classical music, then they might take offense because they assume—through no fault of yours—that you look down on them. This is the key issue: people do crazy things to defend their egos. Many people will assume, from your dietary choices, that you think you are somehow superior to them—not just their food choices, but *them*. They will say the strangest things, and bring up the subject of food around you when it's not even relevant to the conversation. It's as though they're obsessing on the subject even when it's the farthest thing from your mind. (This is most common among people with the worst diets and those who have never met a vegan, which varies greatly depending on which part of the country you typically roam.) Depending on who these people are, and how they behave, this obsessiveness can manifest as anything from genuine curiosity to rude and uninformed challenges to your chosen lifestyle. (Fear not; you will quickly develop responses to handle any situation.)

Some of your peers do not want to admit—especially to themselves—that they might not be making the best choices. Not just for themselves, but for what they feed their families (and that's a whole other set of mega-emotions—*am I being a good parent?*). But the real soul-searching is to be done by you: Do your peers have a low standard for their own health and well-being? Ask yourself that and think about the people you spend most of your discretionary time with. If you choose to spend time with people who don't share similar health values, and if circumstances or personalities are such that this is always an issue, then they can quickly bring you down. And that's not cool.

A recent study shows that behaviors (good or bad) such as healthy eating or smoking pass from friend to friend. People influence one another's health simply through socialization. Therefore, make sure you're influenced in the right direction. Proximity plays a role.

I had some friends in my peer group who were not into healthy living much at all. I had a higher standard for my health than they did, and this bothered them, although it was not something they would admit. They would try to get me to eat like they did because that would validate their lifestyle. This became a problem, and I had to do some real soul searching about whether it was smart for me to hang around these people. Even if I didn't give in, there would always be a slight discord, a lack of harmony in the group. It might have been minor, but it was still negative, and it's not the kind of thing I want to submit myself to for very long.

My health is a priority because it makes everything else in my life better, so I take it very seriously. As a result, I found I had to change my peer group. When you develop a peer group with people who are *doing better than you at the things you value for yourself*, they become an inspiration, rather than a liability. You suddenly have to strive and work harder to keep up with them. It's like the old saying, "Hang around people smarter than you" (so you'll always be getting smarter). Seek out people who live the lifestyle you wish to live and spend time with them. Not only will your new peer group help pull you in the direction you want to go, you'll also learn a lot quickly.

THROW A RAW FOOD PARTY

Your social life does not have to end simply because you now eat raw. Have a fun raw food prep party. One of the reasons people are intimidated by raw food (this includes your family and friends) is because they know nothing about it, such as how to make it, what to eat, and most important, why. One of the best ways to get friends and family involved is to have a party where you teach them how to make raw food (and have them help in the process. It's amazing how much more people like something when they help make it). I find it hard to believe that anyone would turn down an afternoon or evening of eating the healthiest food in the world (maybe with a glass of organic vegan wine). This is a fantastic way to help others learn about raw food. Promise your friends a lot of fun and delicious food to eat.

When I host my raw food prep parties, I pick out four or five recipes for us to prepare. Before the party, I make copies of the recipes and buy all of the ingredients. I tell my friends to bring some containers for leftovers. I serve wine, put on fun music, and have all of my favorite raw food books out for browsing. We have a blast!

Most of all, it gives people a chance to actually *taste* the food! It sounds obvious, but people really have no idea what the heck you're talking about until they try some of these delicious recipes. That's when the lightbulb goes on. Prior to that, they assume you mean veggie platters and boring old salads.

BE PREPARED WHEN PEOPLE OFFER YOU FOOD

Part of succeeding with raw socially is having tactful responses ready when people offer you food. Naturally, you can always say, "Thank you, but I'm vegan," which is fine, but this often invites a conversation that you might not want to have at that moment. If you're not in the mood to go there, here are some good replies to have ready:

* **I just ate a little while ago.** (If you're like me, it's rare that you haven't eaten something—like a piece of fruit—fairly recently.)

* **Thank you, but I'm on a strict regimen of raw fruits and vegetables. Doctor's orders. I'm addicted to sugar (or salt) and I won't be able to have just one, unfortunately. So I have to pass, but thank you.**

* **I brought something for myself so I'm all set, thank you.** (This is a great opportunity to offer them a taste of what you brought.)

Another great method is to ask people to help you achieve your goal, and in the future to not offer cooked foods. Most people—at least, the ones worth hanging out with—will want to help you if you ask them for help. If they can be a part of it, they usually jump at the chance. Tell them you've never been happier or felt better and you don't want to ruin it. This can be very effective with people in your peer group who don't share your health goals. If they're able to support you and help you, even if they don't do it for themselves, this will allow you to stay in the group without constantly having to defend yourself.

The fundamental point here is that it's easy to give in to cravings or peer pressure if you are not prepared. If you have some ready-made responses for when people offer you something, you are setting yourself up to win, like going into battle wearing titanium armor instead of being buck naked. You will find that such rehearsed preparation is less necessary over time because you get stronger as time goes by. Eventually, you'll know how to deftly handle questions, and best of all, the people in your life will get the point.

BEING PREPARED AND EATING OUT

Having prepared food on hand at all times is one of the easiest, most sure-fire ways to succeed in living the raw lifestyle. When you are hungry or want a snack, it's as simple as reaching into your refrigerator. Keep bowls of fresh fruit and raw trail mix on your counter within reach. Just seeing delicious food is motivating and reminds you of your healthy lifestyle.

When you're away from home, it is especially critical to be prepared. Have snacks and food with you at all times. This applies to both short and long outings. I have a little bag that I take with me to restaurants that has a tiny bottle of raw olive oil, a little baggie of sprouted and dehydrated sunflower seeds, my Himalayan crystal salt in a little jar, cayenne pepper, and a few other things. I get lemon wedges from the restaurant, and then I can always dress a salad or plain veggies. Sometimes I even bring a little bottle of my own homemade raw dressing.

Buy yourself a special cooler to use in your car (mine is a medium-size, soft-sided cooler), fill it with ice packs, and put food in it for the day when you go to work, events, family gatherings, and so on. If I'm away from home for even half a day, I pack my cooler with fruit, veggies, seeds/nuts, ice, salad, a green smoothie, and other foods. I can head out without worrying at all that I'll be stuck somewhere and get hungry. You never know when it may happen; you might find yourself in a traffic jam or sitting for a long time in a waiting room. This preparation makes all the difference in the world.

I sometimes call ahead to restaurants, and usually the chef is more than pleased to accommodate my special request for vegan food or a nice raw vegetable and fruit plate. I also have a small laminated card I carry in my wallet that I give to the waiter to show the chef. It reads: "Hello, I eat raw plant-based foods. I'd greatly appreciate it if you could make me a plate with any of the following on it"; then I list a bunch of different fruits, veggies, olives, and so on. This gives the chef an idea of what foods I can eat. And if you do the same and you like what the chef prepared, make sure he or she and the manager know how pleased you are.

A note of caution here, though. Some restaurants won't let you bring in outside food, so if you bring something of your own, do it inconspicuously. I treat my health as if my survival depends on it. Not only am I completely unapologetic about sneaking healthful food into places that don't have the sense to know they should be offering it, but, I'm the *high priestess of food smugglery!*

Some restaurants are more raw-friendly than others. At Mexican restaurants, I order guacamole and salsa, and I might bring my own flax chips or strips of red bell pepper to dip into them. (Tortilla chips are often vegan, but not always, so be sure to ask. But not only are they cooked, they are deep fried, which is very unhealthful if the oil contains trans fats, which are as bad as cholesterol.) At other kinds of restaurants, I typically get a salad (or even two!), or if they have a vegetable side dish, I'll ask to have it raw and order a couple of them. If the chef can't come up with anything better than plain veggies, no problem. Why? Because I came prepared! I squeeze lemon on my salad or vegetables, sprinkle on some of the salt and sunflower seeds that I carry with me, and voilà! It's fantastic.

For family or business outings, the most obvious tip is to eat *before* the event. Otherwise, I try to let people know what to expect of me beforehand. This helps to eliminate any awkwardness if I bring my own dish to a function, meeting, or social time. It's a great conversation starter too, because people always ask me why I eat raw. Moreover, I tend to bring a little extra for others to sample, if they seem interested. This is a good way to spread the word about raw.

If I don't see anything on a restaurant menu I can eat, or I haven't brought my own food to someone's house, I use it as an excuse to relax my digestive system and just drink water or herbal tea. It is not always easy, but it gets easier every time. It becomes empowering to know that you have total control over what goes into your body. I'm always aware that I am only a couple hours away (at the most) from my delicious and healthful raw, organic vegan food. I realize that it might sound extreme to go out to eat at a restaurant and not eat anything, but it's not. Heart surgery is extreme. Cancer is extreme.

Eating well should not be socially awkward. I'm comfortable eating the way I know I should, and I'm happy to explain it to others, but if anybody has a problem with my dietary choices, the bottom line is that it really isn't my problem.

But I almost never experience awkwardness, mostly just sincere questions, which is to be expected. I share these strategies with you to underscore the point that it's not a valid excuse to let social pressure keep you from eating the way you choose to eat. It's funny, but every single argument ever delivered to a teenage kid about peer pressure and alcohol/drugs applies here: just because everybody else is eating crap doesn't mean you should!

FREEZING FOODS CAN BE VERY HELPFUL

One of the ways I make my raw vegan lifestyle easy is by taking advantage of my freezer. By doing this, I make foods in advance and nothing goes to waste.

There are two types of packaging/containers I use for freezing: glass or plastic bags. When I freeze nuts/seeds, nut/seed butters, nut/seed milks, hummus, soups, dried fruit, dips, or dressings, I use mason jars. And, to make the freezing process even better, I use my FoodSaver (as described in Chapter 8, you can buy a separate attachment for mason jars).

When I freeze dehydrated foods such as pizza crusts, crackers, or quiche crusts, or when I freeze desserts or pâté, I usually use FoodSaver bags (yes, they're plastic, but using plastic is necessary for things like quiche crusts, pizza crusts, desserts, and frozen bananas. And, they're BPA-free and made without PVC and phthalates as well). The FoodSaver is great for freezing raw foods! In fact, my mom froze individual slices of my raw vegan cheesecake *over a year ago* using her FoodSaver and sucking out as much air as possible without smashing the dessert. It tasted as delicious and as fresh as the day I made it. Talk about longevity! Heck, get a FoodSaver and make your holiday desserts now! Be prepared and save yourself time during the busy holiday season.

Now, all that talk about the lovely FoodSaver doesn't mean you can't successfully freeze food without one. When I know I'm going to consume something within a month's time or so, for example raw desserts like cookies, chocolates, cheesecakes, and so on, then I just slice it into individual servings (or create the individual cookies or chocolates) and freeze them in mason jars or square glass storage containers, the kind with snap-on tight-sealing lids.

Some raw foods freeze better than others. A good rule of thumb is, the higher the fat content, the better a food usually freezes.

TAKE A BREAK FROM FOOD PREP

You may not always feel like fixing your own food, yet there aren't many great raw choices at restaurants. That's okay, because you can plan ahead for this event not just by freezing foods, but by ordering raw meals from one of the places that ship them nationally. Treat yourself to this once in a while. It will give you a few days' worth of food and you won't have to think about preparing it. The two I know of at the time of this writing (and there may be others) are RAWvolution.com and PureMarketExpress.

SHAKE YOUR BOOTY

Moving the body changes the brain's mental state. Any time you are experiencing a craving or having doubts, don't think big picture (long-term benefits are not as real to the brain as short-term benefits or short-term discomfort). Instead, think about the five minutes *immediately in front of you and get your body moving!*

* Stand up and stretch.
* Breathe deeply.
* Take a walk around the block or even just up and down your street (this one is easy and can be done virtually anywhere, so no excuses!).
* Walk up and down a few flights of stairs if you're in a multistory building.
* Do jumping jacks wherever you are.
* Jump rope for thirty seconds (this sounds like a short amount of time, but it's tough if you're not used to jumping rope, and it feels great!).
* Put a rebounder (mini-trampoline) near your desk (if you have the space) and jump on it like a teenager! Kick those legs out, throw your arms up, and squeal with delight!

GET A PET

Even if it is a goldfish or turtle, a pet is great for helping you focus your attention on something other than yourself and food. Studies have shown that just having a pet nearby makes us feel calm and is, therefore, good for our health. And if you adopt a pet in need of a home, you've done something good not just for yourself, but a fellow creature.

GO RAW WITH A BUDDY OR LOVED ONE

An easy way to succeed in living the raw lifestyle is to do so with a buddy or a loved one. You can test recipes together, exercise together, and share ideas and information. You can buy in bulk, thereby getting a better discount on the food, and divide it between you. You can prepare raw food dishes and have a food exchange, where you make a big batch of a particular recipe and give half to your buddy and vice versa. This helps save time and money, and adds variety to your diet without adding work.

REWARDS IN THE MAIL: REFRESHING YOUR MOMENTUM

This is one of my favorites! It's really fun and exciting to order new things for your new raw lifestyle. Do a little shopping every few weeks, even if it is just to buy a new flavor of flax crackers, a cool organic cotton T-shirt, a new book, a tool for your kitchen, a box of raw food from an online retailer that ships nationally, or some organic hand cream. Because this is not about mindless consumerism, and I strongly advocate trying to live a sustainable lifestyle, don't buy things you don't need or won't use—make sure it's something you'll get value from. You definitely don't need to spend a lot of money. And don't buy your goodies all at once; the idea is to treat yourself to something every few weeks. This gives you something to look forward to, acts as a constant reminder of what you are doing, and *refreshes your momentum.*

TURN TO THE EXPERTS

To improve your health game even more, look to the experts. In the beginning, I bought books, audio CDs, DVDs, and anything I could get my hands on so that I was constantly surrounded by positive and knowledgeable influences (heck, I still do). I read and reread the best books because they continue to teach me and inspire me to be the best I can be. Another great option is to hire a raw coach, and there are plenty available nowadays. These people can help you reach your goals faster than you would on your own, because with a coach, you're accountable. It's amazing what we'll do to live up to somebody else's expectations of us even when we don't always feel like living up to our own.

I continue my education by attending other classes and reading whatever I can get my hands on. It does not stop with classes, community meetups, books, DVDs, and audio CDs; I also attend events, such as potlucks, seminars, and expos with like-minded people. There are lots of raw food events around the world, and you should attend them whenever you can. There are also plenty of retreats and resorts that specialize in raw food, detoxing, cleansing, relaxing, and so on. Consider spending your next vacation at one of those places. Online communities are great, but there's no substitute for the experience of face-to-face interaction with hundreds of people who eat the same way as you; it makes you feel part of a vibrant and thriving community.

GET EDUCATED AND INSPIRED FOR RAW

Surround yourself with this amazing lifestyle. Immerse yourself. Start learning more about it every chance you get, taking full advantage of everything you can get your hands on. Here are a couple of ways to do that.

Read! I get inspired when I flip through a book or magazine about raw food, even if I have already read it (many times!). Simply reminding myself of how others have succeeded with raw is very powerful. I'm drawn to testimonials of people succeeding with raw, so I read these frequently. Another place to look for inspiration is recipe books. I hear this all the time from people who purchase my recipe books, but it works for me too! I'm *constantly* reading my own recipe books to plan and get excited about what I'll be making the following week. It becomes habit-forming!

Watch videos and listen to audios! Following are some DVDs that I highly recommend. They aren't specific to raw food; rather, one covers eating a plant-based diet, for instance, and another discusses genetically modified foods. These DVDs contain a great deal of information, and they reinforce the idea of always being a conscious consumer of food, doing nothing by default or without informed decision-making. I watch these repeatedly. Sometimes I have one of them playing in the background while I'm getting ready in the morning to get my mindset for the day.

Recommended DVDs

* *Forks Over Knives*
* *Food Matters*
* *Eating*
* *The Future of Food*
* *Earthlings*
* *Food, Inc.*
* *A Delicate Balance*

Recommended Books

* *Diet for a New America*, by John Robbins
* *The Food Revolution*, by John Robbins
* *The China Study*, by T. Colin Campbell
* *Skinny Bitch*, by Rory Freedman

After watching the DVDs a few times, you might want to pass them along to somebody else, or better yet, donate them to your library, to help get the word out. I keep mine because I like to watch them from time to time, but I lend them out to people, too. This is democracy in action, true grassroots—the way that fringe ideas start to become mainstream. Tip: Write your name on the case with a Sharpie to make sure you get it back! Or if you give it to someone, make him or her promise to pass it along to someone else.

Take classes! You need to immerse yourself and make your new lifestyle second nature to you. This will accelerate your transition and keep you energized well after the newness has worn off. Sign up for local raw food prep classes and seminars. Even if they focus on basic things you think you already know, you can always learn something new from a different teacher. Students tell me all the time that they love coming to my classes because they find them to be inspiring. Sometimes you even learn from others attending the class. The gathering of students and like-minded individuals with the same goal is powerful. If classes are not offered in your area, start asking for them. Go to local natural foods stores and community education classes at your local community college and leave word that you're interested in classes on raw food preparation. (Then have your friends call and do the same!)

Get online! Check out raw Web sites and join online forums where you can answer other people's questions or get answers to your own questions. Watch YouTube videos of people preparing raw food or talking about how they are succeeding with the raw food lifestyle. Read raw blogs that discuss living the lifestyle. There are many! (Be sure to visit my blog at KristensRaw.com/blog—from there, you can find me on Facebook, too.) Blogs are especially important if you are doing this without the support of your family or friends, because you will connect with other people around the world and realize you are not alone.

COMMUNITY

Another way to surround yourself with like-minded people is through get-togethers, activities, potlucks, and so on in your own community. Check out MeetUp.com, where you will probably find raw, health, and fitness-oriented groups in your local area that you can join. Don't look for raw exclusively; mix it up with people who are vegetarians, vegans, and into alternative health. These are groups that are particularly open-minded to raw. And, don't be afraid to attend these meetings by yourself; in fact, most people usually do. If you can't find a group near you, start one yourself and use MeetUp.com to advertise it.

STOP MINDLESS EATING AND START EATING MINDFULLY

One of my favorite books is *Mindless Eating*, by Brian Wansink, director of the Cornell University Food and Brand Lab in Ithaca, New York. He has been studying the field of food psychology for over twenty years and has made some ground-breaking findings related to people's eating habits. Here's some of what Dr. Wansink has to say about mindless eating: "There are five major areas where people tend to overindulge: dinnertime, snacking, at restaurants, at parties, and desktop/dashboard dining. The music, the number of dinner companions, how long we're sitting at one table—all of these factors affect how much we'll eat."

The solution to mindless eating is to know when to be more mindful about food. Part of the key to succeeding here is to be prepared. Realize before going to a party that you might need to leave the party early or watch how much you're eating and drinking at the dinner table.

When snacking, do not snack from the whole jar. Take out a small portion, put it on a plate, and enjoy. When eating at your desk or in the car, again, portion control will help prevent overeating. Always serve yourself less than you think you might want. If you're still hungry after eating the smaller portion, you can always get more (but there's a good chance you won't). But if you take more at the beginning, you're almost certain to eat it just because it's there. Again, Dr. Wansink: "Our eye judges amounts by using contextual cues, so a helping of mashed potatoes on a 12-inch [30.5-cm] plate, for example, is going to look like less than it would on an 8-inch [20-cm] plate. If you think you're too smart to be fooled, think again."

SOLUTION: Take advantage of this phenomenon by using small bowls and plates. Replace short, wide glasses with tall, skinny ones. A tall glass that holds the same amount of liquid as a short glass makes it seem that it holds more because our brains register tallness more than stoutness when it comes to sizing things up.

WRITE DOWN YOUR FOOD PLAN

One of my favorite things to do each day (after so many years, I still do this) is to write down what I plan to eat the following day. I usually do this at night while I'm lying in bed. I use the "notes" application on my iPhone to write down ideas of what I could eat the following day. I use it as a guide, and this planning keeps me on track.

CLEANSE

"Cleansing" is a broad term that refers to giving your digestive system a rest (thus helping it to detoxify) via a temporary abstinence of food or certain kinds of food. It is also called "fasting." Cleansing, or fasting, means that you restrict what goes in, not that you necessarily stop eating altogether. For instance, you might cleanse by eating only fruit, or by drinking smoothies, juice, or water for a period of time.

Cleanses are a great way to keep you in that motivated "jump start" frame of mind, like the excitement you have when you first go raw. Every few months, I try to do some sort of cleanse, which further cleans me out, gives me extra energy, and makes me love raw food all over again. There's nothing that can make you appreciate a simple tomato or piece of lettuce more than having to restrict yourself from eating for a set period of time. It's like that old saying, "You don't know what you've got until it's gone." Experiencing true hunger, in all its stages, also can have important psychological, spiritual, and social implications—not the least of which is learning not to take anything for granted. (For these and other symbolic reasons, fasting is an important ritual in many religions.)

My cleanses vary, and they typically last from 1 to 3 days. Some people do them much longer—30 days, or even more—but I consider such cleanses to be very advanced and even dangerous for beginners. I do not recommend attempting them without first conducting much research, gaining some experience, and consulting with a doctor who is knowledgeable about and comfortable with the basic idea of cleansing. In fact, you should consult your naturopath or physician before starting any form of cleansing, whether a green juice cleanse, green smoothie cleanse, or fruit cleanse.

REST

True silence is the rest of the mind, and it is to the spirit what sleep is to the body—nourishment and refreshment.
—William Penn

Getting adequate rest is a critical component to well-being and optimal health. And I'm not just referring to sleep. Every day, if possible, you should take five to fifteen minutes to just rest. Rest your eyes. Quiet your mind. Think about the sky, or the sun, or the trees, anything that is calming. Or, think about nothing at all, if you're capable of doing this. If you're not, it's a very important skill to learn, and it's not very hard if you take a quick, one-session introductory meditation class or buy a CD or DVD on the subject.

Take an occasional warm bath; light a candle, soak in some aromatherapy bath salts or oils and just relax. Don't use the time to reflect on the day you just completed or to plan the following day. Just take the time to think about the blue sky, the color of clouds, the fall leaves as they change colors, the ocean and the beach, a bird flying—even the pattern of plaster on the wall—it doesn't matter what; just let it happen. Your life will change remarkably by incorporating these five to fifteen minutes into each day.

Power naps are another fantastic way to get rest and increase your energy, if your routine allows it. Cornell psychologist Dr. James Maas, author of *Power Sleep*, says a 20-minute nap in the afternoon actually provides more rest than sleeping an extra 20 minutes in the morning. Be sure not to nap longer than 30 minutes however, or you may find it difficult to wake.

NEVER GIVE UP

Never give up. This may be your moment for a miracle.
—Greg Anderson

If you fall off the wagon, don't be discouraged! Sometimes the harder you fall, the stronger the momentum you have to get back up. You'll find yourself equipped with an even stronger mind-set that nothing can stop you. Use this to your advantage. Be encouraged. I like what Tony Robbins (the personal-growth expert) says: "When you're frustrated, that is the time to get excited—*because you are about to have a breakthrough*."

I've been there; I know how it can be. There have been times when I fell off the raw lifestyle for part of the day, and since cooked food can have addictive qualities, I would end up finishing the day with even more cooked food. Then, even though I promised myself that on the following day I would go back to raw, I would eat something cooked again. Finally, I would get fed up with mistreating my body, noticing unhealthy and uncomfortable physical changes after only a couple of days or less of being "off" raw, and this motivated me to take back control.

Looking back at the times I went off course, I see that each one became shorter in duration and less severe because I was making better choices over time. The important thing is not how many times you fall off course; rather, if you fall off, how long do you stay off? How quickly can you get back on and learn from it? And, learn you will! You learn more about yourself every time. You make progress, you grow, and you become more proud of your accomplishments. You become stronger every time you do something new or learn new things about yourself, and it empowers you. Don't be discouraged if you slip. Just get right back on the raw path, starting with your *next meal*. You'll know from previous experience how quickly you can rally, meaning you won't be afraid and become demoralized. You'll also start to gather more raw versus non-raw data points and realize that you consistently feel best when you eat raw, and this will help keep you on track in the future.

Any time I went off my raw path, I always got right back on. It might have taken a day or two of reflection to rebound, but I did it. During these reflections I recognized that each time I was actually a little better to myself. One of the first times I went off the raw path I had a vegan burrito, a soy cappuccino, and a vegan cookie (okay, it might have been three cookies)—all in one meal. I'm telling you this because even I—*a raw food chef*—have gone off the path. Each time, I made better choices despite the hiccup. I like what author Tim Ferriss has to say about dieting: "The decent method you follow is better than the perfect method you quit."

I can't emphasize enough the importance of acknowledging your incremental victories. Eventually, you will naturally gravitate back toward raw or high raw, because at some deep level, your mind and body know that's where you belong.

TRAVEL IN THE RAW

Travel happens for many reasons, good and bad. For some people, travel is associated with vacationing, which is supposed to be relaxing and fun. Some people travel for work. Some people have to travel at the last minute due to emergencies. It doesn't matter what the reason is for the travel, people living the raw lifestyle usually have the same concern: How to stay raw while traveling?

Just because you're not in your own kitchen doesn't mean that you can't maintain your awesome raw lifestyle. The key is to be prepared. When going on vacation, if you have the time to plan a few things in advance, your ability to stay raw while you travel will be that much easier. And for those times that you have to pack and leave quickly, it's always nice to have a few things on hand to grab on your way out the door. (While the following section is geared toward travel in the United States, with some adjustment, it could apply to many other developed countries.)

Here are some obvious things to keep in mind. If you're able to get fresh organic food on your trip, then you should bank on that and not pack as much. Just pack enough for the day until you can buy some fresh produce. This applies to trips in the car where you're driving for days or trips where you fly. Check your destination on the Web for locations of Whole Foods, Sprouts, Trader Joe's, Sunflower Market, local farmers' markets, and some of your other favorites that carry organic produce. Then, you can mark them on your map for traveling. I love using apps on my iPhone to facilitate this, such as the Whole Foods Market, VegOut, and Locavore apps. They are fun and useful.

You can also always go online and order fresh organic food to be delivered to your travel destination. It'll cost you a few extra bucks, but it's worth it. Why? Because you're worth it! DiamondOrganics.com or BoxedGreens.com are great places to start, and they'll typically deliver right to your hotel room or wherever you are staying. Also, you can order from places such as BlueMountainOrganics.com or TheRawFoodWorld.com for treats (flax crackers, cookies, and so on), and why not? You're on vacation, right? Spend the extra few bucks to have healthful food shipped to where you're going if you're going to be there for a while. Or, order a few days of raw meals from RAWvolution.com and/or PureMarket Express.com delivered to your destination if you're staying somewhere with a refrigerator or cooler.

And if you're unable to follow any of the following tips, take a memento with you to remind you that you embrace raw. Your memento could be a good luck charm, a raw food book, or anything to remind you that you normally live a lifestyle that is healthy and high in raw food. Then, if possible, use your travel time to relax and not worry about staying raw. Look at your reminder from time to time and say to yourself, "I live a lifestyle high in raw food and nutritional excellence. This is here to remind me of that. While I'm traveling, I might allow myself to have some cooked food and indulgences, but when I'm back home, I'll go right back to embracing raw." And resume *the day* you get back.

Car Trips

Tailor your list of foods and tools for car trips to your specific needs based on the duration of your trip and the number of people you're feeding. The following list will help get you started. If you travel by car frequently, stock a kit with items you'll need so that you're always ready to just add fresh foods and go.

Raw Travel Kit

* A cooler and zip-top plastic bags doubled up with ice to keep the cooler cold (as it melts, dump out the melt-water and refresh it with ice from fast-food restaurants, gas station soda pop machines, or ice machines at your hotel)
* A quick-dry table cover (this really makes any location seem like home, especially if you're in a hotel room, and it's great for picnic-style road trips)
* Wooden plate (or bowl)
* Bamboo flatware
* A small, flexible chopping mat
* A knife with a protective case
* A small rubber spatula
* A vegetable peeler
* A beverage container(s) with watertight lid(s) (filled with water)
* Plastic bags for trash and compost
* A kitchen towel, sponge, biodegradable cleanser (travel size), and a baggie to store sponge between uses
* A lightweight blender such as the Tribest Personal Blender (short trips) or Blendtec blender (long trips)
* Digestive enzymes (supplement) if you end up eating cooked vegan food. These can help you digest the food.
* A protein powder for quick protein shakes to mix with water
* Green powder so you can stay green even if you can't have your fresh green juices and smoothies
* Favorite seasonings and Himalayan crystal salt
* Frozen coconut water or purified water, which serves as ice in the cooler; once it's thawed, you drink it
* Filtered water for food prep (smoothies, soups, rinsing produce)

* Small containers of granola, dried fruit, nuts, and raw snacks
* Apples, pears, Fuyu persimmons, bananas, oranges, grapefruit, lemon, and/or avocados, which don't require refrigeration
* A large baggie of salad mix, washed and ready to eat
* A container of raw salad dressing
* Green smoothie
* Nut milk (or a sprouting bag with a drawstring for sprouting seeds and/or straining nut milk; soak seeds in the sprouting bag inside a zip-top plastic bag filled with water, then remove the sprout bag after 8 hours and hang it to drain)

Airplane Trips

Tailor your list to your specific needs based on the duration of your trip and the number of people you're feeding. The following list will help get you started.

If you're going by plane, you need enough food in your carry-on to get you through the plane ride, plus some things in your luggage to make life more raw-friendly once you've arrived at your destination.

Some of the following can be in your carry-on, and some will have to be in your checked luggage or a separate box. Airplane trips are tricky these day because of the new regulations. The TSA's rules for air travel security are always changing. As such, you may need to make adjustments based on what you are allowed to bring on the airplane with respect to food and liquids.

Raw Travel Kit (split between carry-on and checked luggage)

* A table cover to make it seem as if you're home, especially if you're in a hotel room
* Wooden plate(s) or bowl(s)
* Bamboo flatware
* A vegetable peeler and a kitchen knife with a cover (obviously, this goes in your checked luggage!)
* A small rubber spatula
* A small jar with lid for shaking dressings
* A kitchen towel, sponge, and biodegradable cleanser (travel size, or purchase when you arrive)
* A lightweight blender: Tribest Personal Blender for short trips, or Blendtec blender for long trips
* Digestive enzymes (supplement) if you end up eating cooked vegan food; these can help digest the food
* Protein powder (and a shaker bottle) to mix with water
* Green powder, so you can stay green even if you can't have your fresh green juices and smoothies
* Favorite seasonings and Himalayan crystal salt
* Ready-to-eat foods like prewashed apples (or other firm fruit with skin), cucumbers (I eat these like a giant carrot stick), carrots, celery, small containers of raw trail mix, and raw cookies or brownies

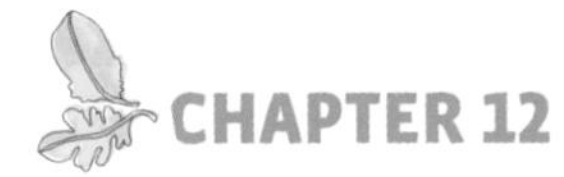

CHAPTER 12

RAW FOOD FREQUENTLY ASKED QUESTIONS

Nothing will benefit human health and increase the chances for survival of life on Earth as much as the evolution to a vegetarian diet.
—Albert Einstein

Here are commonly asked questions and answers about eating a raw diet.

Is Raw Expensive?

No, living the raw lifestyle is not expensive. In the beginning stages, it can *seem* expensive, but in the long run it is definitely not. During the beginning period, when you are new to raw, you might need to acquire some equipment, but that's typically a one-time expense. Initially, you'll also be trying a lot of new recipes and you may not have all of the ingredients on hand, so you will frequently be buying new ingredients as you stock your pantry. Once you're stocked with all the appropriate seasonings, herbs, and ingredients (like raw agave nectar, raw chocolate, raw carob, raw coconut crystals, lecithin, Medjool dates, etc.), you'll only need to purchase them from time to time.

And remember: Living the raw lifestyle means not eating out at restaurants very often. This alone can save you a lot of money. In fact, if you currently eat out frequently, you could save hundreds of dollars each month.

The equipment cost you pay in the beginning can add up, but if you purchase high-quality equipment you won't need to buy these items again (or for a very long time). But reasonably good equipment is available at good prices, so don't let money stop you. Use what you have or buy what you can afford. Later on, you can upgrade your kitchen one piece at a time with higher-quality tools. Ask for these gifts for holidays, birthdays, anniversaries, etc. (I do!)

And remember the things you will *not* be buying, which will save you money. Meat is expensive. Processed and packaged food is expensive. Going to restaurants is expensive. Doctor co-pays and bills are expensive. Prescription drugs are expensive. Being sick and staying home from work is expensive. Not having enough energy to really pay attention to your kids and be there for them 100 percent is expensive.

For some people, the transition to raw can be challenging, due to such stressors and distractions as cravings for cooked food, pressure from outsiders, and advertising galore about the deadly but addictive foods that have made obesity an epidemic in this country. At times, it may almost feel as if you are depriving yourself. To compensate for the mental anguish some people experience, they find themselves trying all kinds of raw stuff, including elaborate and rich recipes (all varied and all needing different ingredients, of course), exotic "super" foods, and so on. It is almost as if people do this to keep their decision justified, or their minds focused to help facilitate their wide-sweeping change in lifestyle. Additionally, you may find yourself making all kinds of food for others to sample, trying to help them understand and support you, or maybe just trying to impress them, or even encouraging them to try the lifestyle for themselves. In this case, there's nothing wrong with alternating simpler with more exotic recipes, both to make meal preparation and entertainment easier and to demonstrate that eating raw doesn't have to involve using all kinds of expensive, unusual ingredients. Eating raw can be quite economical. And the value, in terms of quality of nutritional content per dollar spent, simply can't be beat. It's really an investment in long-term health and quality of life.

No Hot Food? Not Even in Winter?

Let's face it; warm food is nice when your body is uncomfortably cold. But people eat a raw diet all over the world, in all climates. Some people opt for a high-raw diet during cold winter months, while others stay all raw. No matter which path you choose, here are some tips to help:

- **Warm your food in a dehydrator.** Simply place your food in a dehydrator set at 130° to 140°F (54° to 60° C) for 1 to 2 hours.

* **Use warming spices like cayenne pepper, ginger, garlic, etc.** Your body has receptors that tell your brain you're warmer when you eat these!

* **Warm your soup or sauce a little on the stove, but only to a temperature where you can still put your finger in it and hold it there.** If your finger hasn't cooked, neither has your food. Or put it in a warm-water bath.

* **Eat and drink foods at room temperature.** For foods stored in the fridge, take them out in advance to warm up to room temperature before eating. Don't eat or drink cold foods when you're already cold!

* **Exercise!** One of the best and most efficient ways to get your blood circulating is through physical activity. It might take only five or ten pushups or four or five minutes of jumping rope. Plus, this is good for you! You should be doing it anyway!

* **Drink warm herbal tea.** It's not raw, but if it helps warm you up, it's worth it, and it's not bad for you in the way that it's bad to destroy your food's nutritional content through cooking.

* **Dress warmer.** Obvious? It works!

And the most obvious of all? Take a hot bath or shower!

Keep in mind that after you have detoxed, you probably won't have as much trouble keeping warm because your circulation will have improved. (Though this may be offset if you lose weight in the form of fat—but really, are you going to complain if you lose a bunch of fat? No way!)

Will I Have Variety Living the Raw Lifestyle?

Emphatically, *yes*! Having variety in your diet is important so that you don't get bored. After all, it *is* the spice of life. Getting variety into your meals can be as easy as using different produce seasonally, weekly, and even daily. I find that most people crave variety (especially in the beginning stages of going raw) because their minds need it in order to stay motivated and disciplined. This need for variety seems to decrease over time. Raw food comes in many different, amazing forms: lasagna, veggie burgers, granola, nut milk, burritos, pizza, and more. And raw food has global flair. You can enjoy Mexican, Italian, Asian, Indian, and Caribbean flavors, to name just a few. Even if you ultimately settle down to a handful of favorite, easy-to-make staples, there's always something new to keep things lively. I can safely promise you that you'll never run out of things to try.

Should I Take Supplements?

I take a handful of supplements. I don't always take them daily, but I take them often depending on the food I'm consuming at the time and other lifestyle factors like stress, illness, intense exercise, pregnancy, trying to conceive, breastfeeding, traveling, medical procedures, and so on.

My diet provides plenty of nourishing nutrients, but various factors in modern life exacerbate free-radical damage, so I don't shy away from getting a little extra help in the form of supplements. And, until I'm growing all of my own food in my own little utopia paradise, eating an awesome array of just-picked for ultimate freshness, I want those extra supplements as backup. Following are some supplements that you could consider (for more details visit KristensRaw.com/store):

* I believe that people who are still eating a lot of cooked food can benefit from taking an enzyme supplement. I also recommend enzyme supplementation during your transition period, or when circumstances prevent you from having access to raw foods.

* When traveling anywhere unfamiliar (or known to have limited food options), it can help to bring along supplements such as probiotics and enzymes, as well as an antioxidant-rich powder such as raw camu camu wild berry powder, which has a very high concentration of vitamin C. I also bring a green powder supplement (my favorites are Vitamineral Green, Greener Grasses, and Ormus SuperGreens). This way, you continue to get plenty of greens in your diet even while traveling. (These are also great choices if you're recovering from an illness.)

* If you are trying to conceive or are pregnant or breastfeeding, talk with your nutritionist, doctor, or midwife about the nutrients you'll need in your diet, and then assess whether you're meeting those needs. In most cases, even if your diet is excellent, you'll want to supplement with whole-food prenatal vitamins and others.

* Vitamin B_{12} (this is a special case; see below)

* Vegan DHA

* Vitamin K_2 (I get mine from Mercola.com)

* Chlorella tablets as well as wheatgrass tablets for extra quality protein, chlorophyll, and cleansing.

* If you opt to add a calcium supplement to your diet, one brand to check out is Ortho Bone Vegan.

* Probiotics if you're not getting them via fermented foods; I like Ejuva's Moflora.

* Vitamin D if you're not getting enough natural sunshine (you should have your vitamin D level tested annually); according to *The Vitamin D Solution*, vitamin D_2, which is vegan, is just as helpful as vitamin D_3.

Will I Become B_{12} Deficient?

The basic structure of vitamin B_{12} is synthesized by bacteria. Meat-eating humans ingest the vitamin primarily in animal food sources that contain these bacteria. While some plant foods contain B_{12}, these foods are not considered a reliable source and vegans are often advised by nutritionists to take a B_{12} supplement. Interestingly, meat eaters are also advised to supplement B_{12}, due to absorption problems. Gabriel Cousens, M.D., argues that vitamin B_{12} deficiency is typically caused by lack of absorption in the intestinal tract.

Reduced B_{12} levels can also be caused by other reasons. For example, pregnancy and breastfeeding can reduce the B_{12} stores of the mother, making supplementation even more important.

I recommend that you get your B_{12} levels checked annually with a simple blood test. I do this every year, and my numbers have always come back fine. The testing confirms that the supplementation is sufficient.

Should I Eat Sea Vegetables?

Sea veggies can contribute a lot to a raw foods diet: minerals, enzymes, vitamins, protein, fiber, and marine phytochemicals. Sea vegetables contain significant amounts of vitamins, especially the B vitamins. A ⅓-cup (7-g) serving of dulse (a type of seaweed) provides about 10 percent RDA vitamin B_2 (riboflavin) and about 42 percent RDA vitamin B_6. You can find sea veggies at natural foods stores and on the Internet. Some people add sea veggies (dulse, kelp, and so on) to soups, smoothies, and salads, or they use nori sheets to make the popular nori veggie rolls. For those who have a problem with the fishy taste of sea vegetables, I've included a special recipe (Sous-Vide Veggies with Kelp Noodles) just for you in Chapter 18. It is designed to give kelp noodles the flavor and texture of regular cooked pasta.

Where Do You Get Your Protein?

This question is asked so frequently that it has become a groan-inducing cliché among vegans. But to me, it's an important and natural question to ask, because very few Americans were raised with nutritional knowledge beyond the terribly flawed, lobbyist-inspired USDA food pyramid (especially the old-school version, which has been improved a little in recent years). And this ignorance extends to most doctors, I'm sorry to say. Most M.D.s take only a one-semester class in nutrition, if any, which is not enough to get a solid grounding in anything, let alone the nuances of nutrition from 100 percent plant-based diets. (Doctors aren't experts on nutrition; nutritionists are. If you need expert nutritional advice, find one of these highly skilled specialists, preferably one well versed in plant-based nutrition.)

So, where *do* plant eaters get their protein? The answer I like to give is that I get my protein from the same place that elephants, gorillas, and horses get theirs—(pause while it sinks in)—from plants! Yes, you heard right, plants have protein. More specifically, I get my protein from fruits, greens, vegetables, nuts, and seeds. (Notably and deliberately absent from the raw food diet are most grains, not only because they usually need to be cooked, but also because of their relatively low nutrient-to-calorie ratio. This also means you are essentially eating a gluten-free diet.)

Many people talk about the importance of not heating your protein to prevent it from denaturing and coagulating (making it harder to digest). Researchers at the Max Planck Institute found that when protein is consumed in its raw, uncooked state, a person needs only half as much as when protein is eaten after it's been cooked.

People also often ask, what about "complete" proteins? That is, do you get all of the essential amino acids? If you have a varied and balanced plant-based diet, you'll have no problem getting adequate levels of all the essential amino acids. Your body can store amino acids, so it's not necessary to eat foods containing all the essential amino acids in one sitting.

Where Do You Get Your Iron?

Great sources of iron include almonds, dried apricots, beans (for people who still consume some cooked foods), carrots, cherries, persimmons, dandelion greens, dulse, parsley, leafy greens, raisins, prunes, pumpkin seeds, sunflower seeds, and miso—to name just a few.

What Is Miso? Is It Raw?

Miso is a traditional Japanese food that is not raw, but is considered a "living" food. That is, it is metabolically active due to fermentation, thereby giving it many of the same benefits possessed by raw foods.

Miso is a salty paste made from fermented soybeans, grains, and other beans. It can vary in color, which is usually due to the length of fermentation (lighter miso is usually fermented for a shorter period and lighter in taste than the darker varieties). Miso is excellent for digestion, high in protein and nutrition. If you make miso soup, don't boil the water before adding it to the soup or you'll destroy the enzymes. Miso contains protein, vitamin K, zinc, and more.

My all-time favorite source for amazing organic miso products (including non-soy) is South River Miso, available at SouthRiverMiso.com. I can't recommend this brand highly enough. Stock up on it because it essentially has no expiration date and they (usually) offer discounts when you buy over a certain amount. It makes a great gift, too, so the next time you go to a party, bring the host a jar of South River Miso.

What Is Namo Shoyu? What Is Tamari?

Namo shoyu is an unpasteurized soy sauce and, like miso, is considered to be a "living" food. It's very salty, so use it sparingly. An alternative to namo shoyu is tamari (I prefer low-sodium tamari). Both of these are great for adding more flavor to raw food dishes.

What If I Need Chocolate?

No problem! Eat raw chocolate, better known in the raw food world as "cacao nibs." Some say, and I agree, that raw chocolate is the new red wine. And why shouldn't it be? Studies show that raw chocolate is a valuable source of magnesium and antioxidants. David Wolfe, one of the biggest proponents of raw chocolate, believes that it can naturally decrease your appetite and increase your energy. He also claims that raw chocolate contains less than one-twentieth the amount of caffeine found in an equivalent amount of coffee. Chocolate also contains phenylethylamine (PEA), which is what our brains secrete when we fall in love. Need I say more?

What If I'm Addicted to Caffeine?

No problem! Been there, done that when it comes to caffeine. Boy, do I remember the days—working long hours, drinking two to three (!) triple-shot-espresso soy cappuccinos. Yikes! I'm surprised my adrenal glands are even functioning. But I kicked the habit years ago. I was determined to kick the addiction, and I did just that by using all of the following tips and tricks described below. I like variety, so it was fun to change it up with different options. That helped keep me distracted and made it more enjoyable.

* Drink fresh-squeezed orange juice in the morning to give yourself some pure raw energy instead of stimulated energy from caffeine. Yum!

* Chiles: These awesome guys can work wonders for your caffeine addiction because they give you a real rush of endorphins. For the hardcore folks out there, think habanero chiles. If you find those too hot, then start with a milder red pepper and work your way up. The idea here is that it must be hot enough to release endorphins, which are the brain's mechanism for dulling pain. The endorphins tackle two issues for you: (1) providing energy so you don't miss the caffeine; and (2) fighting headaches that may result from caffeine withdrawal. Of course, be careful when handling chiles. Wash your hands when you're done and don't touch your face!

* Drink green juices (lots), including wheatgrass if you like, which helps to alkalize your blood and reduce cravings for caffeine. Add carrot juice, either straight or in the green juice, which will give you an energy boost.

To help avoid severe withdrawal problems, consider cutting off caffeine gradually. You can drink a weaker version of regular coffee, or half caf and half decaf, then eventually work your way to 100 percent decaf.

* Organic tea can rock the house. Both black tea and green tea are reputed to have a number of beneficial health properties, along with a more subtle caffeine boost than coffee. So, it's a great way to enjoy a hot beverage with a little caffeine as you transition away from toxic and often pesticide-ridden caffeine-filled coffee. Yerba maté tea, known as the drink of the gods in South America, is also popular. Its leaves contain vitamins, minerals, amino acids, and antioxidants. And, finally, you can have herbal tea as a goal beverage when you're ready to eliminate all the caffeine in your diet. (My favorite brands are Traditional Medicinals, found at natural foods stores, and Mountain Rose Herbs, found online.) If you like your tea a little sweet, add a touch of raw agave nectar, raw coconut nectar, a pinch of stevia, or a tablespoon of goji berries. Those make an awesome treat to eat at the bottom of the cup when they're nice, plump, and warm.

* If cola, Mountain Dew, Red Bull, Jolt, or some other energy drink is your brand of poison, you'll get a triple-whammy benefit by weaning yourself off of these antithesis-of-healthful beverages. You'll be eliminating not only caffeine, but also (1) a fairly disgusting quantity of sugar (or artificial sweeteners, which bring their own host of problems); and (2) carbonic and phosphoric acids that are bad for your blood, leach calcium from your bones, and dissolve the enamel on your teeth.

As with coffee, it may be easier to reduce your quantity gradually, such as by ordering a medium instead of a large soda, or pouring out the contents of a can when you're two-thirds of the way through. Another great idea is to gradually cut your fountain drinks with soda water when available at self-serve fountains (it's usually dispensed by a little hard-to-see plastic tab that may or may not be labeled). Diluting your caffeine and sugar with soda water won't reduce the acidity, but it will help you taper off caffeine without denying yourself the refreshing and cleansing fizz—what I like to call "throat Drano." Caffeine is much more addictive than bubbles, so once you've kicked your chemical addiction to caffeine, it will be much easier to phase out carbonated beverages entirely.

* Drink Teeccino, which is "herbal coffee." Made from chicory root, it's not coffee at all; it just closely resembles it in color and flavor. My husband and I are big fans of this. For my husband, it was love at first sip. For me, although I really enjoyed it and would drink it here and there years ago when I first stumbled upon it, it wasn't the perfect coffee replacement. I was such a hardcore coffee lover, I didn't think anything would ever compare to the real thing. That being said, here I am, loving Teeccino—big time! Teeccino is much better for your health than regular (or decaf) coffee, and can help transition you away from caffeine. I've even brewed coffee mixed with Teeccino for some of my coffee-addict friends to reduce the caffeine. They love it.

Not only does Teeccino taste great, but it's not acidic so it's safe for pregnancy and breastfeeding. It's high in potassium, helps restore alkalinity, and can help improve digestion. I usually get the Maya Caffe (organic) because it's the most coffee-like in flavor. We love it plain (black), but we also enjoy it with raw nut milk or other nondairy milk for a nice creamy experience. It's brewed like coffee in a coffeepot, but recently the company has launched a new product: Teeccino tea bags. I love this because now I can take it with me to restaurants and enjoy it after a meal.

* Make a beverage (or food) with raw chocolate powder. Raw chocolate has only small amounts of caffeine, but it has a stimulating effect from theobromine. Many people love raw chocolate for the natural buzz they get when consuming it. There are many ways to enjoy raw chocolate powder: (1) Blend raw nut milk with raw chocolate powder and a sweetener until warm for a hot chocolate drink; (2) make chocolate nut milk by adding raw chocolate powder and a couple of pitted dates to the next batch of raw vegan nut milk you prepare; or (3) make other raw food recipes that call for raw chocolate (I have an entire book of raw vegan chocolate recipes; see KristensRaw.com/books). Raw chocolate is satiating, delicious, gives you energy, and is full of antioxidants.

* A great way to start the day is with a cup of warm organic miso soup. You'll be warmed from head to toe, feeling great, and I bet you won't even miss your old cup of joe.

* Set a schedule for yourself. Decide a plan of attack for eliminating coffee from your diet and write it on your calendar. Try the different methods outlined for ease and success, and enjoy the healthy transition. Remember, part of the addiction is the experience associated with consumption (such as going to a cafe or wrapping your hands around a big, warm mug), so look for ways to replicate the experience without the caffeine. Find new places and new cafes and wrap your hands around a big mug of green smoothie, warm herbal tea, or yummy Teeccino.

If you don't want to give up coffee completely but would like to drink it in a more healthful way, I strongly recommend checking out cold-brewed coffee, made with a Toddy Maker. It isn't raw and it still has caffeine, but it's less acidic than regularly brewed coffee, so it's a good way to start (I'm all about the baby steps!). In the scheme of things, cold-brewed is better than regular coffee. Use it as a stepping-stone on your way to eliminating coffee from your life. You can find these machines online at Amazon.com.

Can I Drink Tea?

Tea leaves are not usually raw. Furthermore, if you use hot water, then no, it is not raw. A better alternative is to make "sun tea" by placing water in a jar, adding fresh herbs, and letting the sun brew it.

However, if you don't have time to make sun tea, I think it is perfectly okay to drink packaged herbal teas (especially if you're cold in the winter). In the scope of things, if you are doing all the other aspects of your diet raw, or even most parts, then drinking some organic hot tea (which probably relaxes your mind and makes you feel good) is, in my opinion, worth its weight in therapeutic gold. If you must go without your tea due to fears that the hot water destroyed something, that alone might stress you out and create more angst than just enjoying your tea. Bottom line: Unless you're absolutely committed to living 100 percent raw, then a nice warm cup of tea is your friend.

Can I Drink Wine on a Raw Diet?

Yes; wine is considered raw. (Beer is not.) It's true that alcohol is toxic and basically destroys many cells in its path, including brain cells. That said, not everyone is going to give up alcohol, and if that includes you, then reach for wine the next time you indulge, not only because it's raw, but because it has its own unique phytonutrients with purported health benefits. Just don't overindulge—enjoy a glass, but try to avoid getting tipsy.

Once you go raw, everything in your body and metabolism is more efficient, so expect to feel the effects of alcohol more quickly and strongly, and from smaller amounts of alcohol, as your body will have become very efficient at absorption. You'll want to recalibrate, drinking less than you used to, or more slowly. Until you discover your new lower tolerance for alcohol, be very careful when you drink. And don't drink and drive.

I highly recommend drinking only organic wine that is low in sulfites (or without added sulfites). This is sometimes a point of confusion because sulfites occur naturally even in 100 percent organically produced wine. According to Roger Boulton of UC Davis's Department of Viticulture and Enology (the science of wine and winemaking), even if no sulfur dioxide is added to wine, fermenting yeasts will produce SO_2 from the naturally occurring inorganic sulfates in the grape juice. Thus, says Boulton, it is impossible for any wine to be completely free of sulfur dioxide.

And just because the wine is raw and even organic does not mean it is vegan. Some wines use egg whites or gelatin to give the wine more clarity. If it says "vegan" on the bottle, then you know without a doubt that it is vegan.

Do I Still Have to Drink a Lot of Water?

Water is critical for your body. The great thing about raw fruits and vegetables is that they are rich in water. To stay hydrated, you should still drink water upon waking and between meals. It is true that you tend to drink less water when eating a raw diet because you are getting more water in your foods, as opposed to cooking it out. (All that steam you see coming off of a hot cooked meal is the water your body is supposed to be getting from food itself, just like every other animal on the planet.) A good rule of thumb is to take notice of your urine. It should be very pale in color (almost clear in many cases and quite odorless). If your urine is bright or dark yellow, then you should drink more water.

What Should I Do When There Aren't Many Raw Food Options Available?

My husband and I trained our family well. By now, everyone knows that when we're invited to a function, we'll bring our own food. Or, we'll eat beforehand and simply bring some snacks. While our family fills their plates with monotone-colored foods that usually lack life and nutrients, we fill our plates with vibrant, rainbow-colored foods. It's quite stark, the difference in our plates versus theirs. And, frankly, I love that. Of course, we always get asked questions and many people want to try a bite. I see these situations as opportunities to show others how delicious raw plant-based food can be. I've brought everything to family gatherings from raw pizza to raw lasagna to raw hummus (and dips) with crudités to salads to raw desserts to green smoothies.

I've found that most people want to eat healthfully (at least some of the time); they just lack the knowledge, habits, or discipline to do it. Therefore, when they're given the opportunity to have a tasty, healthful meal that is brought to them (meaning they didn't have to prepare it, and somebody else is providing it), they are usually excited. Even if it's not something they'd normally eat, they still like giving their bodies healthful food when the opportunity arises. And sometimes they're just curious. This explains why raw food restaurants, like Sarma's Pure Food and Wine in New York City, are routinely packed with omnivores! They want an extra-healthful meal once in a while, but they usually want someone else to make it for them, either because it's easier or they think they'll lack the expertise to make it themselves. Too bad they don't know how simple gourmet raw foods can be!

Going to restaurants is a little different, because it can be hard to bring your own food into a dining establishment. Still, I've done it. For example, if we're going to a Mexican restaurant, I'll bring along flax crackers and red bell pepper strips, carrots, celery, and so on, to dip in their salsa and guacamole. Once, we attended a birthday at a bar (greasy bar food, alcohol, etc.), and since I knew ahead of time where we were going, I made a green smoothie and carried it in my purse. I do this all the time. If the wait staff ever challenges me, I say, "I'm on a special diet from my doctor and I can't eat anything grown with pesticides." (This has never failed me—I think the medical aspect scares restaurants in this litigious society.)

Naturally, I don't flaunt my food or drinks, and I generally can avoid confrontation. If it was ever a real problem, I'd leave the food in a cooler in the car, and just go out there a couple of times to snack, if I were that hungry. Again, it's the training of family and friends that matters. They used to think my husband and I were weird, but now they think it's just how we are, and it has become "normal" to them that we live our lives this way. What's even funnier is that now, when they come across someone else eating vegan or raw, they jump at the chance to tell that person that they know someone (us) who eats that way, too.

I've noticed this happening more often in my life, especially now that the health benefits of vegan and raw food have come onto the mainstream media's radar screen. It feels as if a tipping point has been reached. Every time friends or family members tell me they met another vegan or raw fooder, I swear I can almost see in their face that social proof has removed another brick of their defensive wall. An idea that once seemed completely crazy to them now just sounds like any of the other myriad dietary options people have these days. Things like this change slowly—I can remember when restaurants didn't even have nonsmoking sections! One day, I suspect that consumer demand will force most restaurants to offer options that are organic and healthy by raw food standards. Long before then, my lifestyle will have ceased to be so uncommon that people feel compelled to mention it. And certainly it will have lost all sense of controversy or strangeness.

But until that day, what it really boils down to is that, when it comes to my and my family's health, I really don't give a hoot what others think. When I first started the raw lifestyle, I let everyone know, either by e-mail or phone, that I was doing the raw thing. I simply said, "I'm into healthy eating and I'll be bringing my own food to functions. I'm happy to answer any questions you might have. I'm doing this for myself, and my family, because our health is our priority." The reaction? Almost universally, "Okay, cool." No big deal.

My health is my responsibility, not anyone else's. It's up to me to take care of myself. And, truth be told, our lifestyle speaks for itself. Once you've been eating raw for a while, the benefits become evident even to casual observers. Specifically, by a wide margin, my husband and I are the leanest, most physically active, and most fit of anyone in our extended families. If anybody wants to get in my face about our diet, all I need to say is, "It makes it easy to stay in shape" and watch how fast they do one of two things: either (1) back down immediately; or (2) get interested and start asking questions out of genuine curiosity.

One last note: For those times that you don't have food prepared or you're out of town and didn't bring anything or you just don't have the money to have raw food flown in for yourself or you just don't feel like dealing with people's comments, I say that it's very much okay to ease up and eat some cooked food. One of the perks about living the high-raw lifestyle is that, by design, there is wiggle room for social occasions and other situations when your options are limited.

What's All This I Hear About Green Smoothies? Are They Really That Good for Me?

Many people use green smoothies to lose weight, because they help reduce cravings and can replace meals and/or snacks. Green smoothies are satiating because they're loaded with fiber, nutrients, and minerals. Not only that, green smoothies can help reduce cholesterol and steady blood sugar levels. And, if you're craving something sweet, you can drink one of these instead of indulging in something less healthful. You'll be amazed at how satisfying these smoothies are. They're also great for weight loss if you drink one 30 to 60 minutes before a meal. I like to think of them as an appetite suppressant—but a healthful one!

Greens are full of many different nutrients, vitamins, and minerals. The problem with eating greens (especially dark greens) is that they don't always taste great (they can be bitter). But that's not a problem anymore, because with green smoothies, which contain other ingredients that reduce the bitterness, they taste delicious. In fact, kids love them, too! They get excited about drinking something that is "green," and that makes it fun. I like to come up with fun names to make them even more exciting for children (okay, and more fun for *me!*).

When deciding what to put into your green smoothie, consider the following greens as options: spinach, parsley, kale, Swiss chard, celery, arugula, sprouts, cilantro, and romaine lettuce. These vegetables are a great source of quality protein and minerals. Fruit options include berries, apples, pears, bananas, mangoes, pineapple, avocados, persimmons, peaches, and plums. Bananas and mangoes are especially good because of their sweetness, and because their texture helps make the smoothie creamy.

Green smoothies are also great for traveling or running errands. I bring my green smoothie with me! I'll take it to the movies for my snack (hidden in my purse—shhhhh, don't tell the movie police!). When I'm out running errands for the day, I keep one or two in a little soft-sided cooler in my car. This way, if I get hungry or have any cravings, I can drink my green smoothie and be satisfied and full of pure, natural energy.

What Is Nut Milk?

Nut milk is nondairy, plant-based milk made from nuts (or seeds) and is an excellent substitute for animal-based milk.

Nut milk is made by grinding nuts in water, using a high-speed blender, until they're partly liquid. A nut milk bag is a nylon mesh bag used to strain out the pulp, leaving you with extra-smooth milk. I highly recommend doing this for ultimate raw milk results. Nut milk bags aren't cheap, though they are reusable. You can get the same result for less money by using an inexpensive paint strainer bag, available at any hardware store. Cheesecloth also works as a non-synthetic alternative, but it's a little harder to work with and doesn't last long.

What Is Food Combining?

Food combining refers to eating different kinds of foods, separately or together, in such a way as to facilitate digestion. Your body uses different methods to digest different foods. Some of these processes counteract others, so your digestion improves if you eat those foods at different times. It's good to know how to combine foods, especially for people who have digestive challenges.

Here are some basic rules for food combining to get you started. It can be difficult to remember all of the rules and combinations, so if this is something you're interested in, I recommend an iPhone app called Food-Combo. It's a fun app that my husband and his friends developed to help people find good food combinations without having to memorize all of the rules or carry a bunch of charts around when they go grocery shopping.

* With apologies to traditional fruit salad, from now on, eat melons by themselves. Period. If there is one food-combining rule that you should always follow, it's this one. Melons can start to ferment in your digestive system if they're combined with other foods that slow down the digestion of the melons. This can cause discomfort and gas. So, if you're eating melon, eat melon alone. Wait about 20 minutes after your last bite of melon before eating other food. If you've already eaten food prior to wanting melon, wait 2 to 4 hours to enjoy the melon.

* Fruit, in general, digests faster than other foods, so you might want to eat fruit before eating other foods. Specifically, certain fruits combine better with other fruits (acid, sub-acid, and sweet are the different types). I find the specific rules hard to remember. The Food-Combo app is an especially helpful guide to properly pairing fruits.

* Drink liquids between meals, not with meals, because liquids can dilute digestive enzymes and slow digestion.

* Leafy greens pretty much go with everything, including fruit, vegetables, nuts, and seeds (except melons, which, again, you should eat separately).

* When possible, keep fats and fruits separate. This obviously flies in the face of many raw desserts, even many of my own recipes.

But, while mixing them might not be ideal, it's a heck of a lot better than eating a candy bar or a processed dessert, which is not only miscombined, but also filled with fat and sugar. At least raw desserts are filled with phytonutrients, vitamins, minerals, and fiber. Furthermore, most people do fine combining these raw ingredients, but if you have digestive difficulties, consider following this rule and see how you feel.

* For optimal assimilation of vitamins, phytonutrients, and minerals, drink fresh green juices on an empty stomach, or 30 minutes before meals.

The Infamous Salt Question—What Kind to Use?

All life on Earth began in the oceans, so it's no surprise that organisms' cellular fluids chemically resemble seawater. Saltwater in the ocean is "salty" due to many different minerals, not just sodium chloride (table salt). We need these minerals, not coincidentally, in roughly the same proportion that they exist in—guess where?—the ocean! (You've just gotta love Mother Nature.)

When preparing food, I always use sea salt, which you can buy at any natural foods store. Better still is sea salt that was deposited into salt beds before the Industrial Revolution started spewing toxins into the world's waterways. My personal preference is fine Himalayan crystal salt. It's mined high in the mountains from ancient seabeds, has a beautiful pink color, and imparts more than eighty-four essential minerals and trace elements into your diet. You can use either the Himalayan crystal variety or Celtic Sea Salt, but I would highly recommend sticking to at least one of these two. You can find links to buy Himalayan crystal salt at KristensRaw.com/store.

What Is Spirulina?

Spirulina, a freshwater, blue-green algae, is a popular supplement for people trying to get more high-quality protein, B vitamins, and nutrients in their diets. Many people consider spirulina to be a superfood and add it to smoothies and desserts, or sprinkle it on food.

What Is Rejuvelac?

Rejuvelac is a fermented drink made from sprouted grain (traditionally wheat) that is rich in healthy microorganisms. It has a mild, almost lemony-tangy-cheesy flavor that can take getting used to. People often drink a small glass in between meals to facilitate digestion, and some use it in recipes to impart a cheesy flavor to raw food such as soups and dressings. You can add lemon juice to the Rejuvelac to add flavor and help keep the Rejuvelac fresh longer.

What Is the Difference Between Juicing and Blending?

Both juicing and blending are important and very good for you, but in different ways. Juicing extracts the juice from fruits and vegetables and separates it from the plants' pulp (fiber), which is usually discarded, but is sometimes used as an ingredient in recipes. Separating the juice and drinking it in pure form makes it easier to get more nutrition per unit of volume than drinking something that's merely been blended. Juicing can be accomplished either with a juicer or by using a blender and then straining the juice in a nut milk bag to separate out the pulp.

Blending means that you use a blender and drink the whole fruit, including the fiber (and with some fruits, even the peel and seeds) as in a fruit or green smoothie. This helps keep you fuller longer and uses less produce, which can save money.

When you are looking for concentrated nutrients, then juice. When you're hungry or want fiber, blend. Both techniques are good, and I don't recommend one over the other. Make both green juices and green smoothies an important part of your life.

Raw or Not Raw?

Many traditional "health foods" might seem as if they are raw, when in fact they are not. And when it comes to marketing food, the word *raw* does not have a regulated legal definition in the way that, say, *organic* does. Some manufacturers are very specific about selling raw (uncooked) foods, oftentimes marketed specifically to raw fooders like myself and located in a raw food section of stores like Whole Foods Markets. Other manufacturers use the word *raw* on cooked products to indicate that they're unrefined, such as "raw" sugar. And some manufacturers, I suspect, willfully take advantage of this ambiguity in order to sound more healthful than they really are. When in doubt, read the package, as many legitimate manufacturers will specify the maximum heat to which the product has been exposed. When it's still not clear, I often contact the manufacturers directly and ask them.

Here are some foods that often confuse people as to whether they are (or can be eaten) raw.

SPROUTED BREAD

There are several types of "sprouted" breads currently available in natural foods stores. These are usually not raw. My research has indicated that most of these breads are heated at temperatures around 200°F (93°C) or more. If you are not sure, don't shy away from e-mailing or calling the company's number on the package. Alternatively, you can make your own raw sprouted bread.

BULGUR WHEAT

This is commonly used in conventional tabouli recipes. Bulgur wheat is not raw. I use hemp seeds in my tabouli recipe to give it a similar color and texture to bulgur wheat, while keeping the recipe raw.

CORN ON THE COB

You can eat corn raw, right off the cob. It's so good, especially when you buy it from a local farmer.

LENTILS, BEANS, GRAINS

While lentils, beans, and grains need to be cooked, sprouted lentils, beans, and grains are considered raw. Many of them are available already sprouted and ready to eat in natural foods stores. Avoid unsprouted lentils, unsprouted dried beans, and unsprouted grains, unless you plan to cook them.

MAPLE SYRUP

Maple syrup is made from the boiled sap of the maple tree. It is not raw, but some raw recipes still call for it.

NUTRITIONAL YEAST

This is not a raw ingredient but you'll still see it in a lot of raw recipes. Nutritional yeast imparts a delicious cheesy flavor. Neither plant nor animal, it's actually a deactivated fungus that has been grown on molasses in petri dishes, then harvested and pasteurized to kill the yeast. It contains up to 50 percent protein, as well as some important nutrients. People challenged with candida typically tolerate it very well.

Nutritional yeast rarely takes up a significant part of any recipe, so, in my opinion, the fact that it's not raw is not a big deal. Its unique cheesy flavor (both raw and cooked) is very helpful for vegans who miss cheese.

POTATOES

I don't recommend eating uncooked white potatoes, as they can be hard to digest. A good rule of thumb is this: Foods that need to be cooked to make them digestible, palatable, or "safe to eat" should be minimized in your diet. I apply this to sweet potatoes and yams, too, but especially to potatoes because as a "white" starch, they are typically lower in nutrients per unit of calories (especially if the potatoes are peeled).

Because heating starches (when required to make them more digestible) destroys nutrients, eating starchy foods is not ideal and can leave you lacking essential nutrients. In order to eat enough of these to get sufficient nutrition, you then consume too many calories.

RICE WRAPS

These are not raw, but you can fill them with a bunch of delicious raw veggies and sauce during your transition period or when eating a high-raw diet.

TOFU

Tofu is not raw. You can, however, find raw sprouted soybeans in many natural foods stores.

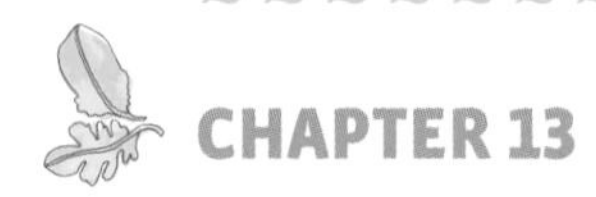

CHAPTER 13

EXERCISE & PHYSICAL FITNESS

A strong body makes the mind strong.
—Thomas Jefferson

No matter how much you're tempted, don't just gloss over this chapter because of its sweaty-sounding title. If you want true health, you won't have it unless you are physically fit. Diet does not make your heart strong, or your muscles or bones strong. Those things require moving your booty and strength training. Without regularly applied resistance, your body literally starts to fall apart.

Diet also does not remove toxins through your lymph system—movement does. The list goes on and on. Even higher brain functions (memory, learning, verbal skills, and so on) have consistently been shown to improve with physical exercise. Some studies demonstrate that physical exercise is more important to brain function than cognitive exercises related to the brain function being measured. In other words, get moving! Note: Always check with a physician before starting a physical program.

If you're not exercising now, why aren't you? Are you waiting for a more ideal time in your life? Um, that would be now. Exercise takes your raw lifestyle to new heights, so get started!

Exercise and physical activity should be an important part of your life—a priority—just like sleeping, eating, drinking water, and resting. It should be a part of your every week, if not every day. If you're frowning at this thought, don't. Exercise is fun and addictive. If you're not already doing it, there will be a point—soon, in fact—when you will crave exercise and physical fitness as a result of eating raw, because the raw lifestyle includes exercise.

Physical activity is not limited to just going to the gym. Exercise can be filled with fun activities like playing with your kids at the park, shopping (lots of walking and carrying bags of purchased goods), walking your dog, dancing, hula-hooping, swimming, jumping rope, and much more.

You will get more out of raw when you add physical fitness to your lifestyle. It is about strengthening your body from the inside out. You'll find yourself with so much energy that you will *want* to exercise. You'll want to get outside and enjoy yourself. As you transition to a high-raw diet, you will find yourself *wanting* to move around. You'll feel so good, you won't be content to just sit on the couch and watch TV. It becomes a virtuous cycle: eating raw food makes you want to work out; working out makes you want to eat more raw! This is how people get sucked into a full-swing raw life cycle and start making dramatic changes in a way that feels totally transformational, yet also seems effortless because your body naturally tells you what to do next.

I have a lot of experience with fitness, strength training, and losing weight. As a former National Physique Committee member, and winner of many bodybuilding trophies, I have learned a lot over the years. According to studies, one session of exercise lowers blood pressure for twenty-four hours. Not only that, exercise will give you a ton of energy and stamina over time. It takes energy to exercise, but as you continue exercising over days and weeks, you build endurance, which in turn gives you more energy on a daily basis, which makes it easier to exercise even more if you want, in another virtuous cycle. This stuff all feeds on itself, so your main concern is just to get the ball rolling, even if that means a simple five-minute walk around the block. After that, your exercise regimen will pick up momentum all by itself. Pretty cool, huh?

I know that not everyone who looks in the mirror feels ready to just "up and get a gym membership." In fact—in the tradition of people who like to straighten up before the housekeeper arrives—some people want to "lose a little weight" before going to the gym. There are, of course, some people who become totally motivated by incorporating intense physical fitness right away, and I love that! (Keep up the great work, because you'll see results much faster if you do.) But, if you lack the motivation, focus primarily on diet first, with moderate exercise, and wait for the virtuous cycle to kick in. The moment you feel the urge to step up your fitness regimen, then pounce on it. You'll know when it feels right. Someday, you'll wake up feeling great, noticing that you feel healthier and are closer to your target weight, and you'll say, "Today I think I'll step things up a bit." And it won't be hard or kick your butt. It will mean that your body has adapted.

Let's keep it real. To be considered truly healthy, you have to be fit. If you are slim, with little or no cellulite and clear glowing skin (this goes for men too!), but you can't make it up three flights of stairs without huffing and puffing, then, I'm sorry, you are not truly healthy. We all know the amazing physical benefits of working out, but there's more. The mental empowerment alone is worth the effort. Studies have shown that one of the best medicines for depression is exercise.

My goal here is to offer you some ways to get started and to get that ever-important little jump-start that gets the momentum and motivation going. If you don't feel like immediately going to the gym, I have included ways for you to start incorporating exercise into your routine today (read: now!) during your regular day, even if it's only on a small scale. This gets the momentum building and gets you excited about exercise and ultimately accustomed to the *habit* of exercise. I am a big believer in baby steps, so here are some tiny things to start doing today (if you are not doing them already). They may seem obvious, but if you are not doing them—then *what the heck are you waiting for?*

* **Take the stairs instead of the elevator every chance you get.** Even if you only have the stamina to walk up one flight and then take the elevator the rest of the way, do it. You will see your strength growing right away, giving you the energy to do more the next time. Don't forget to track your progress. Literally write it down somewhere. It's more fun if you do and it is a powerful way to build momentum.

* **Park in a spot far away from the door to whichever establishment you are headed.** This is probably the easiest way to get extra steps into your day. It's truly a no-brainer, and if you are not doing it already, get to it! As an added benefit, if you park away from other cars, the odds of getting your door dinged drop to almost zero.

* **Take an eight-minute walk two times a day.** That is the approximate length of two of your favorite songs. So, put on your headphones (keep them near you at all times) and listen to two of your favorite *get movin' tunes* and get out there and *walk!* Or jog or whatever, but just move.

* **Set a timer on your cell phone or watch to stand up and stretch every two to three hours.** Once an hour is ideal, but I realize that baby steps are important. If you start with every three hours now, it will not be long until you are doing it more and more often. When you stretch, try to touch your toes, stretch your neck, pull your knees (one at a time) to your chest, reach to the ceiling, etc. Take nice long and deep breaths while you are doing this. It's very effective at helping your circulation and the all-important toxic-removing lymph system, which does its job primarily through *movement* of your body and limbs.

* **Clean the house.** This might seem like a boring chore, but not if you realize that it is good physical activity, too. While you're at it, put on some good music that gives your cleaning a little boogie boost. Not only will you burn a few extra calories, but you'll also start to embed a habit of movement and energy in all that you do—just as children do.

* **Do yard work; in fact, learn to love it.** This follows the same logic as cleaning the house. Yard work can definitely help you burn calories, so get out there and rake leaves, plant flowers, mow the lawn (not a riding mower), or shovel snow and then call it a day because you just accomplished a lot (exercise and chores, simultaneously).

* **Wear ankle weights around the house.** My mom even wears hers to the store, and people always comment that it's a great idea.

* **Dance to your favorite music.** Remember, life is a party—so *dance!*

* **Do sideways leg lifts or calf raises while you're blow-drying your hair.**

* **Do three pushups a day (if you're new to this), or more (if you're not new).** Not girly style, either—no knees on the floor, if you can help it. If you can't do three pushups, then do one or two. You'll gain strength quickly, and you'll find yourself adding extra pushups soon.

* **Get a hula-hoop and hoop during one of your favorite songs every day, for the duration of the whole song.**

* **If you live in a house or building with stairs, when you are watching TV at night, during every commercial break, take the opportunity to go up and down your stairs three to four times (with ankle weights on, if you have them).** If you don't have stairs, then do abdominal crunches for one whole commercial, then do jumping jacks for the next whole commercial and so on and so forth.

* **Get a jump rope.** I cannot tell you enough how amazing jumping rope is. It's one of the highest-calorie-burning activities you can do, and guess what? You burn a ton of calories *in a fraction of the time* you would spend walking or using the elliptical machine or stair-stepper at the gym. It's that intense. In fact, I'll bet that most people reading this right now can't even

jump rope for a minute straight. Try it. It's fun, cheap, and can be done almost anywhere (making it great for traveling).

* **Exercise in the morning.** This really ensures that you do it and don't let "life get in the way." Then, if you have extra time at night, do something else physical (such as the suggestions found in this section). A walk around the block is perfect. It's also a great way to clear your mind, often allowing you to come back to whatever you were doing with renewed focus and alertness. Remember, before we became creatures of cars, phones, mortgages, and nine-to-five servitude, we were creatures of walking, running, gathering food, playing, and dancing. We are fundamentally creatures of *movement*.

* **And speaking of walks, take a ten-minute walk after lunch and/or dinner.** This helps facilitate digestion, too. Robert E. Thayer, a professor of biological psychology at California State University, has found that as little as ten minutes of brisk walking leads to very significant increases in energy throughout the entire day.

* **Take up a new hobby for your spare time in the evening.** This is when a lot of people feel restless, so find something to occupy your time other than just watching TV and snacking. Some great examples are yard work, gardening, playing with your children or pet, dance lessons, music lessons, or art, such as painting, pottery, woodworking, or making things out of stained glass.

* **Watch your posture!** It's very important to stand up straight, sit up straight, and walk with excellent posture. Poor posture can reduce the amount of oxygen you take into your lungs by more than 30 percent. But that's not all. Poor posture affects the way you feel mentally. It affects your mind-set. According to Dr. Rene Cailliet, chairman of the department of physical medicine at the Santa Monica Hospital Center, when you're stooped over you tend to feel old and even depressed sometimes. So sit up straight, shoulders back, and take a deep breath. This can make all the difference in the world!

* **Breathe!** This is one of the simplest and most effective ways to increase your energy and prepare yourself for exercise. You can even do this in your car or at your desk while you're working. Follow these steps:

1. Inhale for a count of two.
2. Hold your breath for four seconds.
3. Exhale for a count of six.
4. Increase these times as you're able.

* **Stay hydrated.** When you are eating a diet full of water-rich fruits and vegetables, you will not need to drink as much water as you used to. However, more is better than less here, so I still drink plenty of water throughout the day. This is especially important when exercising, during the hotter summer months, or if you live in a dry climate. Drinking plenty of water helps keep me energized and alert. When I am looking for an extra little "oomph" of energy, I drink ice water to wake me up.

NOTE: Filtered tap water is just as healthful as bottled, it costs much less, and it is far better on the environment. (Buy bottled water only when there is no alternative.) If you need recommendations on a good water filter, see KristensRaw.com/store. And have fun with it. I sometimes even make my own mint water by adding a stem of mint leaves to a jar of water and letting it soak overnight. Delicious and refreshing!

Nothing great was ever achieved without enthusiasm.
—Ralph Waldo Emerson

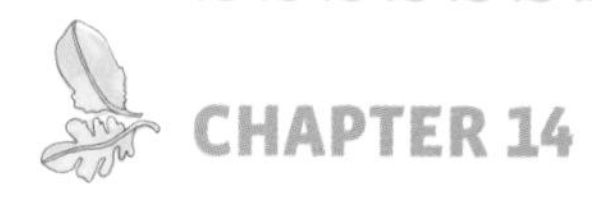

CHAPTER 14

GETTING FAMILY SUPPORT

One of the first questions people ask about going raw is how to get family support. It's actually quite easy (for even the most stubborn families), and this chapter will show you how.

* **Start slowly when you are introducing the idea of raw food to your family.** In fact, it should probably be a slow transition for you, too. Taking your time and using baby steps, whether it's just you that's transitioning or your family too, makes it almost unnoticeable. For example, have smoothies for a couple days; on some other days have raw desserts. Those are both good beginner raw foods that people don't even realize are raw. When I stay at my mom's house, I make Five-Minute Walnut Oatmeal Brownies (page 190). My stepdad loves them and never even asks whether they're raw. They're simply delicious, with a chewy, chocolaty texture and flavor, and he wolfs them down.

* **Involve your family and ask for their support, whether it's for just you or the whole family.** When you ask your family to

support you, it makes them a part of your process and experience. I think it's fundamental that most people *want* to help others. And, when they are asked to support you, it can completely change their mind-set and view of what you are doing. Suddenly the focus is on *you* and not on them. I think that people naturally start looking at their own behavior when someone else is making changes. This can cause problems, because people do not want to admit they are doing anything wrong. So, if you ask them to help you, they don't even realize it but the focus is taken off them and they are more likely to support you. Eventually, as they see the phenomenal health changes in you, they actually want to try it themselves, with no defensiveness because you never confronted their lifestyle. This is one of the best ways for family to get on board—doing so voluntarily—because it usually means a much higher success rate. Here's a sample script of what to say to family and friends:

"I'm trying to feel better and get more energy (or lose weight, or reduce my headaches, etc.), because I really need it. I think adding some healthful fresh foods to my diet might do the trick. But it might be hard because I'm crazy for sugar and processed foods. I'd love to cut some of those out of my diet. Can you help me?"

* **Get your family's opinion and take requests for recipes.** Show your family different raw recipes from books and the Internet, and let them take turns picking out which recipes you make for them to try. Or, ask your family for some of their favorite flavors and pick out something to make based on that. This is especially helpful for kids, because it allows them to make a choice, which gives them ownership in the process. Make it extra fun and have everyone pick two or three recipes each. Write the names of the recipes on scrap pieces of paper. Put them in a bowl or hat and draw one each week. Kids also love helping with recipes. If they help make it, they're much more likely to like the results!

* **Okay, if you know your family won't go for the aforementioned support and ownership stuff, forget all that—*be stealthy!*** Start making one raw dish for every dinner or every other dinner, and don't even mention it. Again, start slowly and add more raw dishes over time—your family probably won't even realize they are eating raw food, just that they will start feeling great! I recommend starting with a raw side dish or soup. (Warm the soup in your dehydrator briefly if that makes it more appealing to your family. If you don't have a dehydrator, you can warm it on the stove on the lowest setting, using your finger to stir it. As long as you can do this, the soup is at a temperature that maintains the integrity of the nutrients and enzymes.)

* **Introduce your family to raw by making a raw dessert.** In no time at all, you'll be having a raw side dish, raw salad with raw dressing, and a raw dessert with every meal.

* **Start preparing big, beautiful salads with vibrant colors and fresh raw salad dressings.** A great way to serve these is on big plates (as opposed to bowls, where foods can fall to the bottom). This way, you can see all of the beautiful fresh produce at once. The best salads, especially for people new to raw, include foods like red bell peppers, olives, raisins, tomatoes, cucumbers, great lettuce, and delicious raw dressing. One trick is to keep the salads simple but vary them every day. So, one night, you might make a salad with red bell peppers, tomatoes, raisins, and olives. The next night, try orange bell peppers, cucumbers, olives, and blueberries or blackberries. Next, make a similar salad but change the lettuce and add chopped pecans or walnuts. Change the dressing every couple of days, too. To add variety, cut the veggies and fruit into different playful shapes such as stars or flowers using inexpensive kitchen tools like cookie cutters and gadgets made specifically for this purpose. Kids notice this even more than adults. (And with kids, it probably goes without saying, anything shaped like dinosaurs is an insta-classic.) By filling up on delicious, huge salads, you and your family will eat much less cooked food.

* **Serve meals in courses.** For example, while you're eating the huge salad, just have the salad on the table. Don't distract your family with bread or crackers or other dishes. This way, they will concentrate on the salad, enjoying all of it and not focusing on anything else. And if they're very hungry, they'll wolf down a lot of it. Then, when everyone is done with the salad, bring out the entree. After everyone is finished, follow with dessert.

* **Start making certain meals raw.** The easiest way to do this is to start making breakfast 100 percent raw. Make fresh organic smoothies for breakfast, or serve plenty of fresh fruit or fresh almond milk with raw granola. Again, it will help if you let your family take part in choosing what flavors to make. So, the night before you make a smoothie, ask your kids (and/or your significant other) which flavors they would like to have. Make it fun by talking about the different colors, too. I love getting my nephews excited about drinking green smoothies. I do this by giving it a much cooler name: "Dragon Smoothies," or "Incredible Hulk Smoothies"—they love that! Or, make a strawberry and banana smoothie and call it the "Barbie Smoothie." Trust me—these things help!

* **And, let's not forget the spectrum from cooked to raw.** Let's say your family typically eats conventional cereal with dairy milk. Start the transition by serving the same cereal but switching the milk to fresh organic raw nut milk. This is a huge step. Ask them which kind of nut milk they'd like (almond, pecan, sesame, walnut, macadamia, hemp, and so on). Find out if they'd like raw chocolate in the nut milk (*yum!*), or maybe some cinnamon and nutmeg. Variety is a key component to success, as is involving your family in the decision making.

* **If any members of your household are active in athletics, urge them to try raw to give them an edge in their game.** This is particularly effective with teens.

* **Here is one of the best ideas (one of my personal favorites):** For every gift you are due to receive (Mother's Day, Father's Day, birthday, holiday, anniversary, and so on) ask that someone's (or your entire family's) gift to you be the gift of him/her/them going raw (or even just vegan) for a set period of time, such as a week or perhaps even a month. Let them know how much this gift would mean to you and thank them every day they're doing it as the best gift ever. This is especially popular with teens and college-age relatives who are short on cash—in my family, they jumped at the offer!

* **Do you need to get your little kids excited to eat more raw fruits and vegetables?** Try this tactic: It's important to give your kids choices so they do not feel forced to eat just one thing. You can do this by offering them something really tasty compared to something that might not be as tasty, thereby making the tasty option seem that much better. For example, offer your kids a choice between blueberries and celery. They will probably pick the blueberries and be happy about it because they had a say in the matter and blueberries taste good (imagine how different this is from offering them blueberries or Oreos!). Or, make it a choice between carrots and zucchini. They'll probably pick the carrots and be happy about it because they got to make a choice. This is an effective way to get more fruits and vegetables in your children's diets.

* **As mentioned previously, another super tip is to cut your children's fruit and veggies into fun shapes and sizes using inexpensive kitchen tools.** (There are entire books about how to make fancy shapes with your produce.) And just imagine how much fun you can have doing this together. Involving your kids in age-appropriate kitchen projects can form not only healthy dietary habits, but also lifelong memories.

* **Include your children in the experience of shopping and preparing food.** This makes them feel more connected to the food, and it makes them feel proud to have helped. When you're proud of something, you tend to want to partake more in it, and children experience the same thing. Have fun while you're doing it and be sure to thank them for their help. I've seen it with my own eyes. When my nephew helps make the food, he wants to eat what he helped prepare. He's full of pride when he does it, and it automatically makes everything taste better to him.

* **Did you know that it's normal to require up to fifteen tries of a new, unfamiliar food before a child likes it?** That's a lot, so don't give up, and don't force it. Just make the food available to try over and over and see what happens. "My child

refuses to eat __________" is often really just a way of saying "my child has more stamina than I do."

* **Eating produce of many different vibrant colors is one of the best ways to ensure that you're getting a broad variety of nutrients, for kids and adults alike.** Here is a great way to get your young children excited about eating naturally colorful, organic foods. Tell them that they get to eat a "rainbow of colors" each day. Get a piece of construction paper for every color of the rainbow: red, orange, yellow, green, blue, and purple. Then, have your children cut out a big, fun shape for each color. On one side of each shape, write the word "DONE" and draw a smiley face. Stick them on the front of your refrigerator door with the word side down. Each day, as your kids eat a fresh fruit or vegetable that is a color of the rainbow, flip over that color's shape so the word "DONE" is faceup. It's a great way to motivate your kids and get them excited about eating all the colors of the rainbow, because they are given a challenge and a sense of accomplishment.

* **Another effective way to get your kids eating more fruits and vegetables is in the form of appetizers.** Family members (kids especially) are usually hungry while you're making dinner, so they ask for snacks. Use this occasion to get more fresh fruit and vegetables into their diets. Always keep a plate of carrot sticks (or other veggies) and fruit available on your counter while you're preparing dinner. Your family will almost always polish off the fruit and vegetables before you're done preparing the meal. A favorite combo in our home is big romaine leaves dipped in Cheezy Hemp Nacho Sauce (page 173). The sauce is so good that people will eat almost anything dipped in it!

* **Kid lunch ideas: Kids love fruit, so give them plenty.** You can also make flax crackers to dip in raw almond butter and sweet berry jam. Raw desserts are also great for kids because they can be eaten any time of the day, and kids love that! Giving your child a piece of raw strawberry pie for lunch is fun and healthy. They also like dipping fresh veggies into raw hummus. You can make many other delicious and nutritious dips for kids that are raw and dairy-free. Best of all, kids love green smoothies because of their cool color. It's an effective way to get more greens into their diets. You can use a few greens (a small handful) at first with plenty of fruit, while the kids get used to them, which is always fast because they taste so great. Let the kids put the ingredients in the blender and push the button. This makes it fun for them. (Make sure they put the lid on first.) Then, get some neat Thermoses to put the smoothies in and send them off to school.

* **Play with your food: Make eating raw food fun.** You already have a head start because of the beautiful bright colors of fresh fruit and vegetables. Now, take it to the next level: make stuff with the food. For example,

make a smiley face out of a salad by using these foods:

HAIR: Spring lettuce mix, sliced cabbage, spinach, or spiralized zucchini

EYES: Grapes, blueberries, olives, or grape tomatoes

LIPS: Red bell pepper slices cut into a smile shape

EARS: Zucchini or cucumber

NOSE: Carrot

Be sure to have some delicious raw veggie dip in a little cup on the side.

Or make a playground:

SWING SET: Asparagus or julienned carrots, with mushrooms as the seats

GRASS: Chopped spinach

MERRY-GO-ROUND: Thick tomato slice

TREES/BUSHES: Broccoli

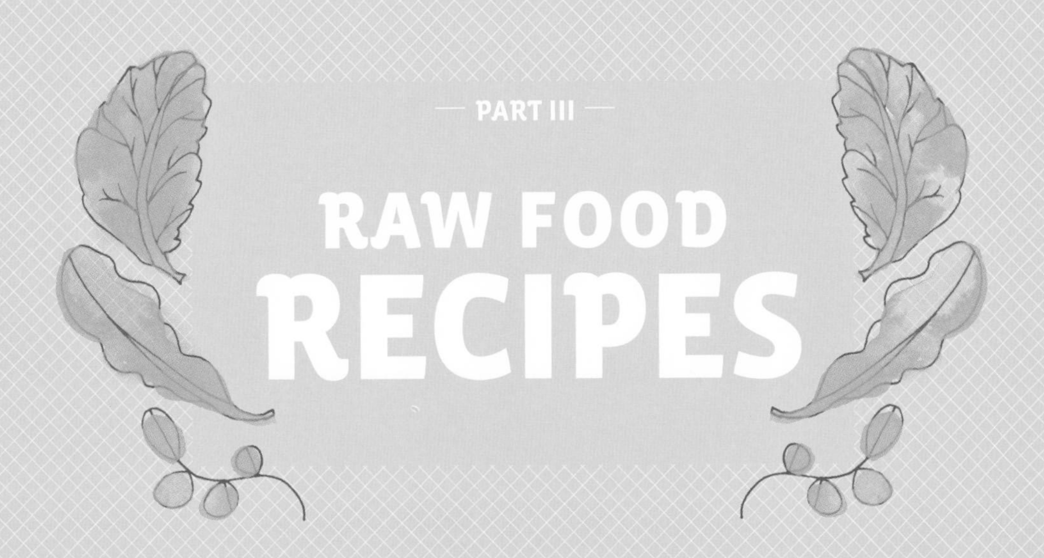

PART III

RAW FOOD RECIPES

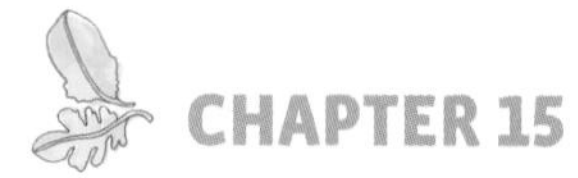

CHAPTER 15

BREAKFAST

CHOCOLATE ALMOND ANYTIME PUDDING

MAKES 4 SERVINGS

I call this Chocolate Almond ANYTIME Pudding because you really can eat it any time. It's full of nutrients and makes a great breakfast, snack, dessert, or pre-workout fuel.

4 MEDJOOL DATES, PITTED
1 AVOCADO, PITTED AND PEELED
1 CUP (240 ML) RAW ALMOND MILK (PAGE 177)
¼ CUP (65 G) RAW ALMOND BUTTER
½ CUP (60 G) RAW CHOCOLATE POWDER
½ TEASPOON ALMOND EXTRACT
PINCH OF HIMALAYAN CRYSTAL SALT
2 TABLESPOONS CHOPPED ALMONDS, FOR SPRINKLING

Place the dates in a bowl and add enough water to cover. Let them soak like this for an hour. Strain off the water and put the dates into a blender. Add the avocado, almond milk, almond butter, chocolate powder, almond extract, and salt and blend until creamy and smooth. Serve immediately sprinkled with almonds. Store leftovers in an airtight glass container in your refrigerator for up to three days. This recipe also freezes wonderfully.

A favorite way that I enjoy this is with sliced banana on top. Additionally, I like to make this so I can have it before a workout, to which I add protein powder. To do that, increase the raw almond milk to 1½ cups (350 ml) and blend in two servings of vegan chocolate protein powder.

BREAKFAST CHIA PUDDING

MAKES 2 SERVINGS

Chia pudding is perfect in the morning because it will keep you full until lunch. Chia seeds are packed with nutrition, including the ever-important omega fatty acids.

1 CUP (240 ML) RAW ALMOND MILK (PAGE 177)
1/4 CUP (35 G) CHIA SEEDS

Put the almond milk and chia seeds in a bowl and stir until mixed. Cover and refrigerate for at least 15 minutes or up to 1 hour before serving.

VARIATION: To add some extra flavor, blend a pinch of stevia, a dash of ground cinnamon, or a drop of your favorite flavor extract into the almond milk before pouring it into the bowl with the chia seeds.

APPLE-PEAR ENERGY

MAKES 1 SERVING

Here is a high-energy breakfast that is easy to make. I'm particularly fond of making this with a green pear and a red apple for the pretty colors.

1/4 CUP (60 ML) RAW ALMOND MILK (PAGE 177) OR WATER
1 PEAR, CORED AND CHOPPED
1 APPLE, CORED AND CHOPPED
2 TEASPOONS RAW COCONUT CRYSTALS OR RAW AGAVE NECTAR
1/2 TEASPOON GROUND ALLSPICE

Put the almond milk, pear, apple, coconut crystals, and allspice in a blender and puree. Serve immediately.

SIMPLE RAW OATMEAL

MAKES 1 SERVING

This recipe is super-fast and -simple, making it a real winner.

½ CUP (45 G) RAW OAT GROATS OR RAW OLD-FASHIONED OATS
½ CUP (120 ML) RAW ALMOND MILK (PAGE 177)
2 TEASPOONS RAW COCONUT CRYSTALS OR RAW AGAVE NECTAR

Put the oats in a bowl and add water to cover by about 1 inch (2.5 cm). Let soak for 8 hours or overnight at room temperature. Drain the oats and give them a quick rinse. Put the oats in a blender with the almond milk and coconut crystals, and blend until pureed. Serve immediately.

CARIBBEAN BREAKFAST OAT GROATS

MAKES 2 SERVINGS

This is a great way to start the morning and get your day going with a bang!

½ CUP (45 G) RAW OAT GROATS OR RAW OLD-FASHIONED OATS
1 CUP (240 ML) RAW ALMOND MILK (PAGE 177)
1 MANGO, PEELED, PITTED, AND CHOPPED
1 BANANA, PEELED AND CHOPPED
¼ TEASPOON GROUND CINNAMON
PINCH OF HIMALAYAN CRYSTAL SALT (OPTIONAL)

Put the oats in a small bowl and add water to cover by about 1 inch (2.5 cm). Let soak for 8 hours or overnight at room temperature. Drain the oats and give them a quick rinse. Put the oats in a blender with the almond milk, mango, banana, cinnamon, and salt and blend until pureed.

SPICED APRICOT-DATE GRANOLA

MAKES 2½ QUARTS (1 KG)

Making your own raw granola is rewarding. In spite of the soaking, sprouting, and dehydrating times (all things that don't actually require much effort on your part), the recipe is easy and fun to make. You will save a lot of money by making your own raw granola, too. It's a perfect excuse to buy a dehydrator if you don't have one already, because it pays for itself quickly when you add up the savings on making your own granolas, crackers, snacks, etc.

1½ CUPS (125 G) RAW BUCKWHEAT GROATS
1½ CUPS (170 G) RAW ALMONDS
1 CUP (120 G) DRIED APRICOTS
10 MEDJOOL DATES, PITTED
1 TABLESPOON CHINESE FIVE-SPICE POWDER
⅛ TEASPOON HIMALAYAN CRYSTAL SALT
½ CUP (70 G) HEMP SEEDS

Rinse the buckwheat groats and put them in a medium bowl. Add water to cover by about 1 inch (2.5 cm). Let soak at room temperature for 12 hours. Drain the buckwheat groats, rinse them, and put them in a colander set over a bowl (to catch the water) with a paper towel laid gently on top of the colander. Allow the buckwheat groats to sprout for at least 12 or up to 24 hours.

When the buckwheat groats are starting to sprout, put the almonds in a medium bowl and add water to cover by about 1 inch (2.5 cm). Let soak at room temperature for at least 12 or up to 24 hours.

About 1 hour before the groats and nuts are done soaking, put the dried apricots and dates in a medium bowl. Add just enough water to cover and let soak at room temperature for at least 30 or up to 60 minutes. Drain, reserving the soaking water.

Put the soaked apricots and dates into a blender and add enough of the reserved soaking water to get the mixture going. Add the five-spice powder and salt. Blend until smooth (add a little extra water if needed).

Drain and rinse the buckwheat groats and put them in a large bowl. Drain, rinse, and chop the almonds. Add the almonds to the bowl with the buckwheat groats. Transfer the blended date mixture to the bowl and add the hemp seeds. Stir until the date sauce coats everything well.

Transfer half the mixture onto each of two dehydrator trays lined with a nonstick Para-Flexx sheet or parchment paper. Spread the mixture out using an offset spatula (the thinner you spread it, the faster it dehydrates).

Dehydrate at 130°F (54°C) for 1 hour. Turn the dehydrator down to 105°F (40°C) and continue dehydrating for 10 to 12 hours. Flip the granola onto two unlined trays and peel off the Para-Flexx sheets. Continue dehydrating for 12 to 24 hours longer, or until you reach the texture you desire.

When dehydrated thoroughly, the granola will keep for up to 2 months.

SPROUTED PROTEIN BARS

MAKES 12 BARS

These are fantastic! They hit the spot for an energizing and nourishing breakfast (or a snack any time of the day). You can toss one in a baggie and take it on the go, too. Sprouted Protein Bars are full of nutrition with their sprouted grains, hemp seeds and chia seeds (essential fatty acids anyone?), and almonds and pecans. I'll take one of these over a store-bought protein bar any day.

½ CUP (90 G) QUINOA
½ CUP (45 G) RAW BUCKWHEAT GROATS
1 CUP (115 G) RAW ALMONDS
1 CUP (115 G) RAW PECANS
½ CUP (60 G) DRIED PAPAYA, MANGO, APPLES, OR APRICOTS
16 MEDJOOL DATES, PITTED AND CHOPPED
¼ CUP (35 G) HEMP SEEDS
¼ CUP (35 G) CHIA SEEDS
1 TEASPOON RAW VANILLA POWDER
2 PINCHES OF HIMALAYAN CRYSTAL SALT
1 TEASPOON FRESH LIME JUICE
⅛ TEASPOON STEVIA (OPTIONAL)

Rinse the quinoa well and put it in a small bowl. Add water to cover by 1 inch (2.5 cm). Let soak for 12 hours at room temperature. Drain and rinse. Put the quinoa in a colander set over a bowl (to catch the water), with a paper towel laid gently on top of the colander. Allow the quinoa to sprout.

Rinse the buckwheat groats and put them in a medium bowl. Add water to cover by about 1 inch (2.5 cm). Let soak at room temperature for 12 hours. Drain the buckwheat groats, rinse them, and put them in a colander set over a bowl (to catch the water) with a paper towel laid gently on top of the colander. Allow the buckwheat groats to sprout for at least 12 or up to 24 hours.

Put the almonds and pecans in separate medium bowls and add water to cover by about 1 inch (2.5 cm). Let soak at room temperature for 12 hours.

About 1 hour before the grains and nuts are done soaking, put the dried fruit in a small bowl and add water to cover by about ½ inch (12 mm) and let it soak to soften.

Give a final rinse to the quinoa and buckwheat groats. Then, put them in a food processor. Drain and rinse the almonds and pecans and add them to the food processor. Drain the dried fruit (reserve the soaking water in case you need it later) and add it to the food processor. Add all the hemp seeds, chia seeds, vanilla powder, salt, lemon juice, and stevia (if using) and process the mixture until blended (at this point you can add some of the soaking water if needed). You might need to stop the processing to scrape down the sides of the bowl a couple of times.

Spread the mixture onto a dehydrator tray lined with a nonstick ParaFlexx sheet or parchment paper. Place some parchment paper on top and use a rolling pin to help spread out the mixture. Remove the parchment paper and score the bars into the desired size.

Dehydrate the bars at 130°F (54°C) for 45 minutes. Turn the dehydrator down to 105°F (40°C) and continue dehydrating for 6 to 8 hours. Flip the protein bars onto an unlined tray and peel off the ParaFlexx sheet. Continue dehydrating another 12 to 24 hours, or until you reach the texture you desire.

When dehydrated thoroughly, the bars will keep for up to 2 months.

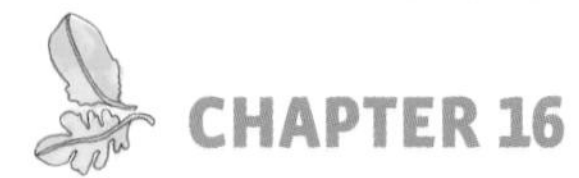

CHAPTER 16

SOUPS

BOUNTIFUL VEGGIE SOUP

MAKES 6 CUPS (1.4 L)

This is a spin-off from my very popular recipe, Kristen Suzanne's Harvest Soup. I love the simplicity of the whole vegetables (and non-sweet fruits), and the cayenne adds a kick of warmth. Feel free to experiment and add fresh herbs for extra seasoning and flair.

½ CUP (130 G) RAW CASHEW BUTTER (PAGE 175)
1¾ CUPS (420 ML) WATER
2 CUPS (240 G) CHOPPED ZUCCHINI
2 TOMATOES, CHOPPED
1 CUP (100 G) CHOPPED CELERY
1¼ CUPS (160 G) CHOPPED CARROT
1 LARGE DRIED TURKISH FIG (SEE NOTE), OR 2 MEDJOOL DATES, PITTED
1 GARLIC CLOVE
1 TABLESPOON MINCED SHALLOT
1 TEASPOON HIMALAYAN CRYSTAL SALT
1 TEASPOON FRESH LEMON JUICE
¼ TEASPOON CAYENNE PEPPER

Put the cashew butter, water, zucchini, tomatoes, celery, carrot, fig, garlic, shallot, salt, lemon juice, and cayenne in a blender. Blend until creamy. (I prefer this soup a tad warm and very creamy, so I blend it for about 2 minutes.) Serve immediately.

NOTE: Turkish figs are absolutely amazing and completely different from the figs you usually see in the store. I get mine at BlueMountainOrganics.com. Each one is a little piece of heaven: large, plump, sweet, and delicious.

CREAM OF TOMATO SOUP

MAKES 3 CUPS (720 ML)

One of the recipes I missed when I went raw was cream of tomato soup. I have wonderful memories of enjoying the traditional version as a child. Coming up with a raw vegan substitute was something I had to do.

When I first created this, I was delighted at how fresh it was, as well as how much better it was than the old cooked stuff I used to eat. As with most of my raw soups, I like to blend this one until it reaches a warm (but not hot) temperature.

1/2 CUP (55 G) RAW CASHEWS
2 CUPS (300 G) CHOPPED TOMATOES
1 CUP (120 G) PEELED AND CHOPPED ZUCCHINI
1 1/4 CUPS (300 ML) RAW ALMOND MILK (PAGE 177)
3 TABLESPOONS SUN-DRIED TOMATO POWDER (SEE NOTE)
2 MEDJOOL DATES, PITTED
3/4 TEASPOON HIMALAYAN CRYSTAL SALT
1/8 TEASPOON FRESHLY GROUND PEPPER

Put the cashews in a bowl and add water to cover by about 1 inch (2.5 cm). Let soak at room temperature for 1 to 2 hours.

Drain the cashews, rinse, and put them in a blender. Add the tomatoes, zucchini, almond milk, sun-dried tomato powder, dates, salt, and pepper. Blend until creamy. Serve immediately.

SUN-DRIED TOMATO POWDER: Simply grind sun-dried tomatoes to a powder in a blender or coffee grinder. One cup (110 g) of sun-dried tomatoes should yield about 3 tablespoons of powder.

CITRUS-CAULIFLOWER SOUP

MAKES 3½ CUPS (840 ML)

Cauliflower is one of those vegetables that I don't long for. However, it's full of nutrients, so I find enjoyable ways to get it in my diet. Enter Citrus-Cauliflower Soup.

2 CUPS (200 G) CHOPPED CAULIFLOWER FLORETS
2 CUPS (240 G) CHOPPED ZUCCHINI
1 CUP (240 ML) FRESH ORANGE JUICE
½ CUP (55 G) RAW PINE NUTS
1 MEDJOOL DATE, PITTED
3 TABLESPOONS FRESH LEMON JUICE
1 TEASPOON CHOPPED GARLIC
½ TEASPOON PACKED GRATED ORANGE ZEST
¼ TEASPOON HIMALAYAN CRYSTAL SALT

Put the cauliflower, zucchini, orange juice, pine nuts, date, lemon juice, garlic, orange zest, and salt in a blender. Blend until creamy. Serve immediately.

INDIAN MANGO SOUP

MAKES 3½ CUPS (830 ML)

This soup is divine! It's creamy, lightly sweet, and packed with nutrition (vitamin C, iron, fiber, folate, vitamin B_6, copper, vitamin K, potassium, and more).

1¼ CUPS (300 ML) WATER
2 CUPS (340 G) CHOPPED MANGO
2 CUPS (60 G) GENTLY PACKED SPINACH
½ AVOCADO, PITTED AND PEELED
1 TEASPOON FRESH LEMON JUICE
¾ TEASPOON GROUND CARDAMOM
½ TEASPOON GROUND GINGER
PINCH OF HIMALAYAN CRYSTAL SALT (OR MORE)

Put the water, mango, spinach, avocado, lemon juice, cardamom, ginger, and salt in a blender. Blend until creamy. Serve immediately.

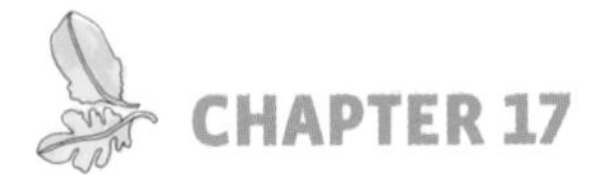

CHAPTER 17

SALADS

PINE NUT–CRUSTED TOMATO SLICES

MAKES 2 TO 3 SERVINGS

Want a super-easy but satisfying salad or snack? Make these!

1/4 CUP (25 G) RAW PINE NUTS
3 LEAVES FRESH BASIL, CHOPPED
1/4 TEASPOON HIMALAYAN CRYSTAL SALT
DASH OF FRESHLY GROUND PEPPER
3 TOMATOES

Put the pine nuts, basil, salt, and pepper in a food processor and process to a coarse consistency. Cut the tomatoes into 1/4-inch-(6-mm-) thick slices. Sprinkle the pine nut mixture on top of the sliced tomatoes. Serve immediately.

STRAWBERRY–LEMON ZEST CREAM OVER APPLES AND BANANAS

MAKES 4 SERVINGS

This recipe's gorgeous pink color, creamy texture, and bright flavor take fruit to a whole new level. Serve this salad for breakfast, lunch, or dessert! And, although I like keeping it easy by making it with apples and bananas, you'll love the cream with any fresh fruit.

CREAM
1 CUP (115 G) RAW CASHEWS
5 STRAWBERRIES
3 TABLESPOONS WATER
5 TABLESPOONS (75 ML) FRESH LEMON JUICE
1 TABLESPOON GRATED LEMON ZEST
1 TABLESPOON RAW AGAVE NECTAR
1/2 TEASPOON HIMALAYAN CRYSTAL SALT

SALAD
4 MEDIUM TO LARGE APPLES, CORED AND CHOPPED
4 MEDIUM TO LARGE BANANAS, PEELED AND SLICED

FOR THE CREAM: Put the cashews in a medium bowl and add water to cover by about 1 inch (2.5 cm). Let soak at room temperature for 1 to 2 hours. Drain, rinse, and put them in a blender. Add the strawberries, water, lemon juice, lemon zest, agave nectar, and salt. Blend until creamy. (Store in an airtight glass container for up to 5 days.)

FOR THE SALAD: Put the apples and bananas in a large bowl.

Add one cup (240 ml) of the cream. Stir well and serve.

BANANA-ROMAINE SALAD WITH GINGER-SHALLOT DRESSING

MAKES 4 SERVINGS

This dressing has a gorgeous flavor and is especially wonderful paired with romaine and banana. Yes, banana—it's not just for green smoothies, you know.

DRESSING

5 TABLESPOONS (75 ML) RAW OLIVE OIL
3 TABLESPOONS APPLE CIDER VINEGAR
2 TABLESPOONS WATER
2 TABLESPOONS RAW AGAVE NECTAR
1 TABLESPOON PLUS ½ TEASPOON TAMARI
1 TABLESPOON MINCED SHALLOT, OR 1 TEASPOON ONION POWDER
1 TABLESPOON GRATED FRESH GINGER, OR 1 TEASPOON GROUND GINGER
⅛ TEASPOON FRESHLY GROUND PEPPER

SALAD

LEAVES FROM 1 BUNCH ROMAINE LETTUCE, CHOPPED
4 BANANAS, PEELED AND CUT INTO ¼-INCH-(6-MM-) THICK SLICES

FOR THE DRESSING: In a blender, combine the olive oil, vinegar, water, agave nectar, tamari, shallot, ginger, and pepper. Blend until creamy.

FOR THE SALAD: Place the romaine lettuce on plates and top with the sliced bananas.

Pour the desired amount of dressing on each salad and serve.

CITRUS WALNUT KALE SALAD

MAKES 2 LARGE SERVINGS

Kale is a staple in our house because of its powerful nutrient profile. Having it in a salad with citrus is a great way to ensure that your body properly absorbs the iron the kale offers.

1 LARGE BUNCH CURLY KALE
2 TABLESPOONS RAW OLIVE OIL
2 TABLESPOONS FRESH LEMON OR LIME JUICE
½ TEASPOON HIMALAYAN CRYSTAL SALT
½ CUP (55 G) CHOPPED RAW WALNUTS
2 TO 3 TEASPOONS MINCED SHALLOT
1 GRAPEFRUIT, PEELED, SEEDED, AND CHOPPED
2 ORANGES, PEELED, SEEDED, AND CHOPPED

Remove the stems from the kale. (You can leave the more tender parts of the stem, toward the top of each leaf, in the salad, but the harder stems toward the bottom of each leaf should be removed.) Tear or chop the kale leaves into bite-size pieces.

Put the kale into a large bowl. Add the olive oil, lemon juice, and salt. Massage all of these ingredients together with your hands. Add the walnuts, shallot, grapefruit, and oranges. Gently toss to mix before serving.

ALMOND BUTTER COLESLAW

MAKES 4 TO 6 SERVINGS

Crunchy cabbage paired with sweet oranges and creamy dressing makes a unique and delicious salad.

DRESSING

3/4 CUP (180 ML) RAW ALMOND MILK (PAGE 177)
1/2 CUP (130 G) RAW ALMOND BUTTER
2 TABLESPOONS COCONUT VINEGAR OR APPLE CIDER VINEGAR
1/2 TEASPOON HIMALAYAN CRYSTAL SALT
DASH OF FRESHLY GROUND PEPPER

SALAD

1 HEAD RED CABBAGE, CORED AND CHOPPED OR SHREDDED
2 TOMATOES, CHOPPED
4 ORANGES, PEELED, SEEDED, AND CHOPPED
1 HANDFUL RAISINS
7 OLIVES, PITTED AND CHOPPED

FOR THE DRESSING: In a blender, combine the almond milk, almond butter, vinegar, salt, and pepper. Blend until smooth.

FOR THE SALAD: In a large bowl, combine the cabbage, tomatoes, oranges, raisins, and olives and toss to mix.

Add the dressing and toss until the dressing coats the salad ingredients. Serve immediately.

FOUR-INGREDIENT MAGIC DRESSING

MAKES 2/3 CUP (165 ML)

This is one of my favorite dressings. It's easy. It's mega-delicious. And, it makes you want to beg for more salad practically every time. While it's amazing on just about any salad, my favorite combo is romaine lettuce, thinly sliced carrots, chopped cucumbers, raisins, red cabbage, and red or orange bell pepper. To make the perfect salad, put your salad ingredients of choice in one big bowl. Pour the dressing on top, then toss the salad well until the dressing coats it all.

1/4 CUP (65 G) RAW CASHEW BUTTER (PAGE 175)
1/4 CUP (60 ML) WATER
2 TABLESPOONS COCONUT VINEGAR (SEE NOTE)
1 1/2 TABLESPOONS TAMARI

In a blender, combine the cashew butter, water, vinegar, and tamari. Blend until creamy.

Store the dressing in an airtight glass container in the refrigerator for up to 5 days.

NOTE: You may substitute the coconut vinegar with fresh lime juice, fresh lemon juice, or apple cider vinegar. All variations are delicious, but my favorite is the coconut vinegar (check out CoconutSecrets.com).

SIXTY-SECOND RAW RANCH DRESSING

MAKES 1½ CUPS (360 ML)

This dressing, from my book Kristen Suzanne's EASY Raw Vegan Transition Recipes, *is so-called because it is easy and quick to make (okay, so maybe it takes some people two minutes to whip it up instead of one minute, but you get the point—it's really fast!). And, more important, it is plate-lickin' awesome.*

Once this dressing is refrigerated, it thickens. At this point, it is still thin enough to use on a salad, but you can always water it down if you like. You can also use the thickened version as a luscious, flavorful dip for veggies.

¾ CUP (180 ML) WATER
½ CUP (130 G) RAW CASHEW BUTTER (PAGE 175)
1 TABLESPOON DRIED DILL
1 TABLESPOON FRESH LEMON JUICE
1 TEASPOON ONION POWDER
½ TEASPOON HIMALAYAN CRYSTAL SALT
PINCH OF FRESHLY GROUND PEPPER

In a blender, combine the water, cashew butter, dill, lemon juice, onion powder, salt, and pepper. Blend until smooth.

Store the dressing in an airtight glass container in the refrigerator for up to 5 days.

OLIVE-TAHINI DRESSING

MAKES ⅔ CUP (160 ML)

Olives and tahini are a wonderful combination, and this dressing will surely satisfy your palette. Enjoy it on any green leafy salad such as romaine, spinach, or arugula.

¼ CUP (60 ML) WATER
¼ CUP (65 G) RAW TAHINI
5 OLIVES, PITTED
1 TABLESPOON FRESH LEMON JUICE
PINCH OF HIMALAYAN CRYSTAL SALT
PINCH OF FRESHLY GROUND PEPPER

In a blender, combine the water, tahini, olives, and lemon juice. Blend until smooth. Season with salt and pepper.

Store the dressing in an airtight glass container in the refrigerator for up to 5 days.

SWEET CURRY-ORANGE DRESSING

MAKES 2/3 CUP (160 ML)

Take a trip to India with these delicious flavors. This dressing will add pizzazz to your next salad. Try it with romaine lettuce, carrots, tomato, and apple.

3 TABLESPOONS RAW CASHEW BUTTER (PAGE 175)
3 TABLESPOONS WATER
1 ORANGE, PEELED, SEEDED, AND CHOPPED
1 1/2 TEASPOONS TAMARI
1/2 TEASPOON GROUND CURRY POWDER
JUICE OF 1/2 LIME

In a blender, combine the cashew butter, water, orange, tamari, curry powder, and lime juice. Blend until creamy.

Store the dressing in an airtight glass container in the refrigerator for up to 5 days.

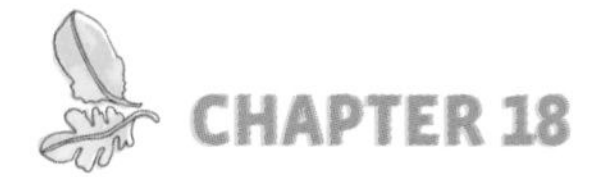

CHAPTER 18

ENTREES

SOUS-VIDE VEGGIES WITH KELP NOODLES

MAKES 2 SERVINGS

This recipe uses three pieces of kitchen equipment: a blender to make the sauce, a FoodSaver to facilitate the marinating and softening of ingredients, and a dehydrator to help marinate and warm the recipe. If you don't have a FoodSaver or dehydrator, simply eat this dish right after it's made (the veggies and noodles will have a firm texture). Or, put the mixture in a large zip-top bag, push out the air, and put it in a bowl of warm water that you keep changing out to maintain a warm temperature.

ONE 12-OUNCE (340-G) PACKAGE KELP NOODLES
JUICE OF 1/2 LIME
2 CUPS (180 G) CHOPPED BROCCOLI FLORETS
3/4 CUP (90 G) THINLY SLICED CARROT
1/2 CUP (25 G) THINLY SLICED FENNEL BULB
1/4 CUP (4 G) CHOPPED FRESH CILANTRO, OR 2 TABLESPOONS CHOPPED FRESH BASIL
2 TABLESPOONS RAISINS

SAUCE

1/2 CUP (120 ML) WATER
1/2 CUP (130 G) RAW CASHEW BUTTER (PAGE 175)
1 TABLESPOON FRESH LIME JUICE
1 TABLESPOON NUTRITIONAL YEAST
3/4 TEASPOON ONION POWDER
1/4 TEASPOON HIMALAYAN CRYSTAL SALT
DASH OF FRESHLY GROUND PEPPER

2 TABLESPOONS CHOPPED RAW ALMONDS FOR GARNISH

Rinse the kelp noodles well and put in a medium bowl. Squeeze the lime juice over the noodles and add enough water to cover. Set aside for 1 hour at room temperature.

Drain the noodles, rinse them, and put them in a large bowl. Add the broccoli, carrot, fennel bulb, cilantro, and raisins and set aside.

FOR THE SAUCE: In a blender, combine the water, cashew butter, lime juice, yeast, onion powder, salt, and pepper. Blend until smooth.

Pour over the noodles and veggies and toss to coat. Put the mixture in a FoodSaver bag and follow the manufacturer's instructions for removing the air. Put the bag in your dehydrator for 1 hour at 135°F (57°C). Reduce the temperature to 115°F (45°C) for another 30 to 60 minutes.

Divide the noodles and veggies between two plates and top with the almonds. Serve immediately.

HERB-AVOCADO KELP NOODLES

MAKES 2 SERVINGS

This dish reminds me of a fresh garden, and the kelp noodles are a fun alternative to zucchini noodles.

ONE 12-OUNCE (340-G) PACKAGE KELP NOODLES
JUICE OF 1 LEMON

SAUCE
1 AVOCADO, PITTED AND PEELED
1/2 CUP (120 ML) WATER
1 TEASPOON MINCED SHALLOT
3 MEDIUM-LARGE LEAVES FRESH BASIL
1/2 TEASPOON CHOPPED FRESH ROSEMARY
1 TEASPOON FRESH LIME JUICE
1/8 TEASPOON HIMALAYAN CRYSTAL SALT
FRESHLY GROUND PEPPER
1/2 TOMATO, DICED

Rinse the kelp noodles well and put in a medium bowl. Squeeze the lemon juice over the noodles. Add water to just cover the noodles. Let soak at room temperature for 1 hour. Drain, rinse well, and return to the bowl. Set aside.

FOR THE SAUCE: In a blender, combine the avocado, water, shallot, basil, rosemary, lime juice, and salt. Blend until smooth. Season with pepper.

Pour the sauce over the kelp noodles and toss until all of the noodles are well coated. Divide the noodles between two bowls and top with the diced tomato. Serve immediately.

OLIVE AND VEGGIE PASTA

MAKES 2 SERVINGS

The first time I made this, both my husband and I knew it'd become a regular in our house. The textures and flavors are refreshing and delicious.

1 LARGE ZUCCHINI
1 MEDIUM TO LARGE RED BELL PEPPER, SEEDED AND DICED
1 AVOCADO, PITTED, PEELED, AND DICED
4 RAW OLIVES, PITTED AND CHOPPED
3 LARGE LEAVES FRESH BASIL, CHOPPED
1 TEASPOON MINCED FRESH CHIVES
1 TEASPOON FRESH LEMON OR LIME JUICE
PINCH OF FRESHLY GROUND PEPPER

Using a spiral vegetable slicer, spiralize the zucchini into noodles. If you don't have a spiral slicer, use a vegetable peeler to cut the zucchini into long, thin slices.

Put the zucchini in a bowl and add the bell pepper, avocado, olives, basil, chives, lemon juice, and pepper. Toss well and serve.

SIX-MINUTE LASAGNA STACK

MAKES 1 SERVING

When you have a craving for hearty lasagna, make this raw recipe. It's super-fast and the fresh flavors will explode in your mouth.

¼ CUP PLUS 2 TABLESPOONS (30G) RAW PINE NUTS
3 LEAVES FRESH BASIL, CHOPPED
2 TABLESPOONS WATER
⅛ TEASPOON HIMALAYAN CRYSTAL SALT
PINCH OF GROUND NUTMEG
2 TOMATOES, CUT INTO ¼-INCH- (6-MM-) THICK SLICES
1 ZUCCHINI, CUT INTO ⅛-INCH- (3-MM) THICK SLICES

Using a food processor, process the pine nuts, basil, water, salt, and nutmeg to a thick puree.

Overlap some of the tomatoes in a circle on a plate. Spread with some of the pine nut mixture. Overlap the zucchini slices on top. Spread with the remaining pine nut mixture and top with the remaining tomato slices.

EASY STUFFED PEPPERS

MAKES 2 SERVINGS

Apart from the soaking time of the nutrient-rich sunflower seeds, this recipe can be whipped up in no time flat. It makes eating raw easy!

¾ CUP (100 G) RAW SUNFLOWER SEEDS
½ CUP (50 G) CHOPPED CELERY
2 TABLESPOONS FLAX MEAL
1½ TEASPOONS MINCED FRESH CHIVES
1 TEASPOON FRESH LIME JUICE
¼ TEASPOON HIMALAYAN CRYSTAL SALT
¼ TEASPOON GARLIC POWDER
⅛ TEASPOON CHIPOTLE POWDER
DASH OF FRESHLY GROUND PEPPER
2 MEDIUM TO LARGE RED, ORANGE, OR YELLOW BELL PEPPERS

Put the sunflower seeds in a bowl and add water to cover by about 1 inch (2.5 cm). Let soak at room temperature for 6 to 8 hours. Drain the sunflower seeds and rinse.

In a food processor, combine the sunflower seeds with celery, flax meal, chives, lime juice, salt, garlic powder, and pepper. Briefly process to a slightly coarse texture.

Cut the top off each bell pepper, including the stem, and pull out the seeds. Stuff the bell peppers with the sunflower seed mixture. Serve immediately.

ALL-STAR COLLARD WRAPS WITH CHILI CREAM

MAKES 2 WRAPS

Using collard greens for a wrap is hardcore. Consider yourself badass. The following recipe lists some of my favorite ingredients for wraps, but don't let this limit you. Instead, let it inspire you. Feel free to swap out the ingredients for other foods in your refrigerator, and let your creative juices flow.

2 LARGE COLLARD LEAVES
1/2 CUP (130 G) CHILI CREAM (FACING PAGE)
4 OLIVES, PITTED AND CHOPPED
1 TOMATO, CHOPPED
1 CUP (55 G) ROMAINE LETTUCE, CHOPPED
1/2 CUP (25 G) SPROUTS
3 LEAVES FRESH BASIL, CHOPPED
1 CARROT, SHREDDED
2 TEASPOONS COCONUT VINEGAR
HIMALAYAN CRYSTAL SALT
FRESHLY GROUND PEPPER

Put the collard leaves on a cutting board and cut off the stems. Score the inner stems horizontally to make the leaves flexible enough to use as wraps.

Spread half of the cream on each collard leaf. Top each leaf with half of the olives, tomato, lettuce, sprouts, basil, carrot, and vinegar. Season with salt and pepper.

Fold the sides of a leaf inward and then roll the leaf away from you. Use toothpicks to help hold it together. Cut the wrap in half with a sharp knife. Repeat with the second leaf and serve.

CHILI CREAM

MAKES 1½ CUPS (380 G)

¼ CUP (30 G) SUN-DRIED TOMATOES
1 CUP (120 G) CHOPPED ZUCCHINI
⅔ CUP (170 G) RAW CASHEW BUTTER (PAGE 175)
¼ CUP (4 G) GENTLY PACKED FRESH CILANTRO
2 TABLESPOONS MINCED RED SERRANO PEPPER
1 TABLESPOON FRESH LEMON JUICE
1 TABLESPOON TAMARI
1 TEASPOON CHILI POWDER
1 TABLESPOON CHOPPED GREEN ONION (GREEN PARTS ONLY)
¼ TEASPOON MINCED GARLIC
⅛ TEASPOON CHIPOTLE POWDER

Put the sun-dried tomatoes in a bowl with water to cover. Let soak at room temperature for 15 to 20 minutes. Drain, reserving the soaking water in case you need it later.

Put the sun-dried tomatoes in a blender and add zucchini, cashew butter, cilantro, ¼ cup (60 ml) water, serrano, lemon juice, tamari, chili powder, green onion, garlic, and chipotle powder. Blend until smooth (adding some of the reserved soaking water, if necessary).

Store the cream in an airtight glass container in the refrigerator for up to 5 days.

PIZZA BITES WITH GARLIC-SHALLOT CHEESE

MAKES 2 SERVINGS

These are fun, delicious, and seriously full of flavor. Perfect as a dinner or lunch. When you have raw crackers (they act as the pizza crust) on hand, it makes for a super-easy entree to throw together.

GARLIC-SHALLOT CHEESE (PAGE 168)
6 TO 8 RAW CRACKERS OR MORE, DEPENDING ON SIZE (SEE NOTE)
1 TOMATO, SEEDED AND DICED
4 TO 6 OLIVES, PITTED AND CHOPPED
3 TO 4 TABLESPOONS CHOPPED FRESH BASIL

Spread the cheese on the crackers. Top with the tomato, olives, and basil and serve.

NOTE: You can buy raw crackers at the store or make your own (see Mexican Crackers, page 172).

GARLIC-SHALLOT CHEESE

MAKES 1 CUP (235 G)

1 CUP (115 G) RAW CASHEWS OR RAW PINE NUTS
1 TABLESPOON FRESH LEMON OR LIME JUICE
1 TEASPOON MISO
2 TEASPOONS MINCED SHALLOT
½ TEASPOON MINCED GARLIC
¼ TEASPOON HIMALAYAN CRYSTAL SALT

Put the cashews in a bowl and add water to cover by about 1 inch (2.5 cm). Let soak at room temperature for 1 to 2 hours.

Drain the cashews, rinse them, and put in a blender. Add the lemon juice, miso, shallot, garlic, salt, and ½ cup (120 ml) water. Blend until smooth. You might need to stop and scrape down the sides of the blender container a few times to facilitate blending.

CHAPTER 19

SIDE DISHES & SNACKS

CUCUMBER GARLIC CHEESE BOATS

MAKES 2 SERVINGS

These make a wonderful lunch, snack, or side dish. The first time I served them to my family, they squealed in delight! My husband said they were criminally delicious.

The cheese sauce is amazing in other dishes as well. You can use it as a dip for veggies, a spread for raw crackers, or a raw pasta sauce over zucchini noodles, and for those of you who aren't all raw yet, it makes an awesome sauce for cooked pasta, toast, and veggie burgers.

GARLIC CHEESE

1 CUP (115 G) RAW CASHEWS
1/4 CUP (17 G) NUTRITIONAL YEAST
1 TABLESPOON FRESH LEMON JUICE
1 TABLESPOON CHOPPED FRESH GARLIC
1/2 TEASPOON HIMALAYAN CRYSTAL SALT

BOATS

2 CUCUMBERS
1/2 CUP (80 G) FINELY CHOPPED RED BELL PEPPER

FOR THE CHEESE: Put the cashews in a bowl and add water to cover by 1 inch (2.5 cm). Let the cashews soak at room temperature for 1 to 2 hours.

Drain the cashews, rinse them, and put them in a blender. Add the yeast, lemon juice, garlic, salt, and 1/2 cup (120 ml) water. Blend until creamy.

Halve the cucumbers crosswise and then slice each half lengthwise. With a spoon, scoop out the seeds and discard. Stuff the boats with the cheese and top with the red bell pepper. Serve immediately.

GARLIC ALMOND–SAUCED BROCCOLI

MAKES 2 SERVINGS

Raw broccoli has never been a passion of mine, so for me, the trick is to serve it with a delectable sauce such as this one. In fact, this sauce is amazing with almost any veggies. My whole family routinely uses it as a salad dressing and fights over who gets to lick the blender clean. It's that good.

2/3 CUP (170 G) RAW ALMOND BUTTER
1/2 CUP (120 ML) WATER
3 TABLESPOONS RAW COCONUT NECTAR OR RAW AGAVE NECTAR
3 TABLESPOONS FRESH LEMON OR LIME JUICE
2 TABLESPOONS TAMARI
3 GARLIC CLOVES
4 CUPS (360 G) CHOPPED BROCCOLI FLORETS

In a blender, combine the almond butter, water, coconut nectar, lemon juice, tamari, and garlic. Blend until smooth. Pour the mixture over the broccoli. Toss until the broccoli is well coated with the sauce and serve.

TOMATO-ORANGE SALSA WITH MEXICAN CRACKERS

MAKES 2 SERVINGS

This combination is so good, and it makes a perfect hearty snack, a light lunch, or an impressive appetizer for the next party you host.

SALSA
3/4 CUP (170 G) DICED ORANGE
3/4 CUP (110 G) DICED TOMATO
1 TEASPOON MINCED SHALLOT
1 TABLESPOON CHOPPED FRESH BASIL
PINCH OF HIMALAYAN CRYSTAL SALT
PINCH OF FRESHLY GROUND PEPPER

4 TO 6 TABLESPOONS (65 TO 100 G) RAW ALMOND BUTTER
6 TO 8 MEXICAN CRACKERS (PAGE 172)

FOR THE SALSA: Toss orange, tomato, shallot, basil, salt, and pepper together in a bowl.

Spread the almond butter on the crackers. Top the crackers with the salsa before serving.

MEXICAN CRACKERS

MAKES 12 TO 16 CRACKERS

These crackers are amazing, and my entire family is crazy for them. The flavors are fresh and vibrant. We love them so much that they were instrumental in inspiring my purchase of a bigger food processor so I could make double batches.

1 CUP (135 G) RAW SUNFLOWER SEEDS
1 CUP (135 G) RAW PUMPKIN SEEDS
2 CUPS (240 G) CHOPPED ZUCCHINI
1 CUP (150 G) CHOPPED TOMATO
1 CUP (100 G) CHOPPED CELERY
½ BUNCH FRESH CILANTRO, INCLUDING STEMS
1 SMALL SHALLOT, CHOPPED
1 TABLESPOON CHILI POWDER
½ TEASPOON HIMALAYAN CRYSTAL SALT
½ TEASPOON GROUND CUMIN
JUICE OF 1 LEMON

Put the sunflower seeds and pumpkin seeds in a large bowl and add water to cover by about 1 inch (2.5 cm). Let soak at room temperature for 6 to 8 hours.

Drain the seeds, rinse them, and put them in a food processor. Add the zucchini, tomato, celery, cilantro, shallot, chili powder, salt, cumin, lemon juice, and ½ cup (120 ml) water and process to a puree.

Spread the mixture onto a dehydrator tray lined with a ParaFlexx sheet or parchment paper. Score the crackers into the desired size and shape. Dehydrate for 1 hour at 130° to 140°F (54° to 60°C). Reduce the temperature to 105° to 110°F (40° to 43°C) and dehydrate another 8 to 10 hours. Transfer the crackers to an unlined dehydrator tray and dehydrate until they reach the level of crispiness you desire (9 to 12 hours longer).

When dehydrated thoroughly, the crackers will keep for up to 2 months.

CHEEZY HEMP NACHO SAUCE

MAKES ABOUT 1½ CUPS (360 ML)

This is one of my all-time best recipes. It has made the Internet rounds, and the feedback is phenomenal. It's approved of, coveted, devoured, and obsessed over by herbivores and omnivores alike!

⅓ CUP (80 ML) WATER
1 GARLIC CLOVE
2 TABLESPOONS FRESH LEMON JUICE
1 RED BELL PEPPER, SEEDED AND CHOPPED
1 CUP (140 G) HEMP SEEDS
2½ TABLESPOONS NUTRITIONAL YEAST
1 TABLESPOON CHILI POWDER (SEE NOTE)
2 TEASPOONS TAMARI
½ TEASPOON HIMALAYAN CRYSTAL SALT
½ TEASPOON GARLIC POWDER
¼ TEASPOON CAYENNE PEPPER
⅛ TEASPOON GROUND TURMERIC

In a blender, combine the water, garlic, lemon juice, bell pepper, hemp seeds, yeast, chili powder, tamari, salt, garlic powder, cayenne, and turmeric. Blend until creamy.

Store the sauce in an airtight glass container in the refrigerator for up to 5 days.

NOTE: My favorite brand of chili powder is Simply Organic.

SERVING SUGGESTIONS

* Dip veggies or corn chips into this (raw or not—it's up to you!). This also makes a delicious dressing on a hearty salad of romaine lettuce, tomatoes, and cucumbers.
* For those eating cooked foods, this is an awesome sauce on top of veggie burgers.
* Use this sauce to make nutritious cheesy-flavored kale chips (see page 174).

CHEEZY HEMP NACHO KALE CHIPS

MAKES 3 TO 4 SERVINGS

Kale chips are great for snacking when you're watching TV, going to the movies, or any time.

1 BUNCH KALE, STEMMED

CHEEZY HEMP NACHO SAUCE (PAGE 173)

Tear the kale into large bite-size pieces (you can use curly kale or dark kale—they both work great—and I usually leave the central stem in, but you can take it out). Put the torn kale in a large bowl and pour the sauce on top. Stir it all up with a big spoon, or your hands, until the kale is covered well with sauce.

Place the kale on a dehydrator tray lined with a ParaFlexx sheet or parchment paper. Dehydrate for an hour at 130° to 140°F (54° to 60°C). Reduce the temperature to 105° to 110°F (40° to 43°C) and dehydrate another 7 to 9 hours. Transfer the kale chips to an unlined dehydrator tray and dehydrate for another 7 to 10 hours, or until it reaches the texture you desire (flexible or crispy).

When dehydrated thoroughly, the chips will keep for up to 1 month.

GINGER-GARLIC SPREAD

MAKES 1 CUP (250 G)

This creamy, nutritious, and flavorful recipe is perfect for dipping all of your vegetables. One of my favorite ways to eat this is with carrots and broccoli. Yum!

1 CUP (115 G) RAW CASHEWS OR RAW PINE NUTS

1 TABLESPOON GRATED FRESH GINGER

1 TEASPOON FRESH LIME JUICE

3/4 TEASPOON MINCED GARLIC

1/2 TEASPOON HIMALAYAN CRYSTAL SALT

Put the cashews in a small bowl and add water to cover by about 1 inch (2.5 cm). Let soak at room temperature for 1 to 2 hours.

Drain the cashews, rinse them, and put them in your blender. Add the ginger, lime juice, 1/2 cup (120 ml) water, garlic, and salt. Blend until creamy.

Store the spread in an airtight glass container in the refrigerator for up to 5 days.

RAWK STAR GREEN HUMMUS

MAKES 1½ CUPS (350 MG)

This is a fantastic hummus recipe. In the past I've made raw hummus that isn't green (making it look more like traditional hummus), but that requires peeling the zucchini, which is where a lot of the zucchini's nutrition is. I prefer green hummus for both the gorgeous color and the nutrition.

2 CUPS (240 G) CHOPPED AND PACKED ZUCCHINI
½ CUP (130 G) RAW TAHINI
1 TABLESPOON APPLE CIDER VINEGAR
2 TABLESPOONS FRESH LEMON JUICE
1 TEASPOON GRATED LEMON ZEST
¾ TEASPOON HIMALAYAN CRYSTAL SALT
½ TEASPOON MINCED GARLIC
½ TEASPOON CUMIN SEEDS
½ TEASPOON CORIANDER SEEDS
⅛ TEASPOON FRESHLY GROUND PEPPER

In a blender or food processor, combine the zucchini, tahini, vinegar, lemon juice, lemon zest, salt, garlic, cumin seeds, coriander seeds, and pepper. Blend until creamy.

Store the hummus in an airtight glass container in the refrigerator for up to 5 days.

RAW CASHEW BUTTER

MAKES 2 CUPS (520 G)

You can buy raw cashew butter pre-made from a store or online, but making your own is rewarding and saves money. I stock up on raw cashews (usually 5 pounds /2.3 kg at a time) so that I'm never without them and I can make raw cashew butter whenever I need it.

4 CUPS (460 G) RAW CASHEWS

In a food processor, process the cashews until they form a paste. This could take 4 to 8 minutes, depending on the food processor. You will likely need to stop the food processor a few times to scrape down the sides and make sure the butter doesn't overheat.

Store the butter in an airtight glass container in the refrigerator for up to 1 month.

VARIATIONS: Use this recipe to make any nut or seed butter: hemp seed, pumpkin seed, sunflower seed, pine nut, Brazil nut, almond, pecan, walnut, hazelnut, pistachio, and so on. The time to process may vary, depending on the nuts or seeds.

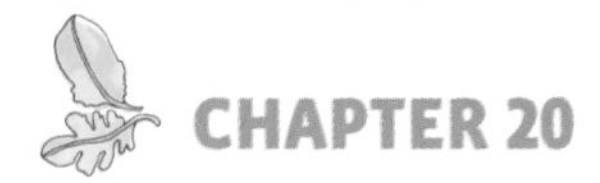

CHAPTER 20

BEVERAGES

RAW ALMOND MILK

MAKES 4 CUPS (1 L)

This is a staple in my refrigerator, and I highly recommend you make it a staple in yours. This almond milk is wonderful and nutritious and can be used in many ways, from drinking on its own to adding to raw granola, blending into smoothies or dressings, and more. I would estimate that I make this one or two times a week, I use that much. You can also make nut milk with other nuts or seeds; see the variations at the end of the recipe.

1 CUP (115 G) RAW ALMONDS

1/2 TEASPOON RAW VANILLA POWDER

SPLASH OF ALMOND EXTRACT (OPTIONAL)

Put the almonds in a medium bowl and add water to cover by about 1 inch (2.5 cm). Let the almonds soak for 12 hours at room temperature. Drain the almonds, rinse them, and put in a blender. Add 4 cups (2 L) water, the vanilla powder, and almond extract (if using) and blend for 1 minute.

If desired, pour the mixture through a nut milk bag to strain the milk and make it smooth. Store in an airtight glass container in the refrigerator for up to 5 days.

VARIATION: You can also make raw vegan milk using Brazil nuts, pecans, macadamia nuts, cashews, hazelnuts, pistachios, walnuts, pine nuts, pumpkin seeds, or sunflower seeds. Just follow the recipe and replace the almonds with your choice of nut or seed. Most nuts and seeds don't need to soak as long as almonds, so you can reduce the soaking time to 6 hours.

You can also make raw hemp seed milk, but for that you don't need to soak the hemp seeds; just blend them with the other ingredients.

NOTE: Most nuts and seeds are not as naturally sweet as almonds so you might consider adding a little sweetener, such as raw agave nectar or yacón syrup; soaked dates, prunes, or raisins; or raw coconut nectar or raw coconut crystals.

For an amazing source of truly raw nuts, seeds, and dried fruits, I recommend BlueMountain Organics.com. Keep in mind that if you buy in bulk, you get a better price.

If you need almond milk but don't have time to soak the nuts, blend 1 cup (240 ml) water with 1 tablespoon raw almond butter. Voilà! Sixty-second raw almond milk!

BERRY-MINT MILK

MAKES 2 SERVINGS

I almost named this Antiaging Mint Milk, because the ingredients are loaded with antiaging nutrients. Whatever you call it, this drink of berries and almond milk is awesome for helping to slow the signs of aging.

1½ CUPS (360 ML) RAW ALMOND MILK (PAGE 177)
1½ CUPS (220 G) BLACKBERRIES
1½ CUPS (230 G) RASPBERRIES
1 CUP (150 G) BLUEBERRIES
1 HANDFUL ICE
2 TABLESPOONS FRESH MINT LEAVES
2 DASHES OF STEVIA

In a blender, combine the almond milk, blackberries, raspberries, blueberries, ice, mint, and stevia. Blend until smooth. Serve immediately.

GREEN SNACK SMOOTHIE

MAKES 1 SERVING

Sometimes I just want a little something to snack on that will hold me over between meals. Enter Green Snack Smoothie. It's easy to make, tasty, and fits the "I need a snack" bill.

1¼ CUPS (300 ML) WATER
1 STALK CELERY, HALVED
1 LARGE LEAF SWISS CHARD, HALVED
2 SMALL TO MEDIUM BANANAS, PEELED AND CHOPPED
1 HANDFUL ICE

In a blender, combine the water, celery, Swiss chard, bananas, and ice. Blend until smooth. Serve immediately.

ORGANIC GREEN SMOOTHIE

MAKES 1 SERVING

Green smoothies are a wonderful addition to anyone's lifestyle. They are a great way to start eating cleaner and get tons of energy right away. If your smoothie tastes too "green," simply add more fruit (or use fewer greens next time). You'll find yourself adding more greens over time because your taste adjusts and your body loves getting the greens, so you end up craving them.

1 TO 2 CUPS (240 TO 480 ML) FILTERED OR SPRING WATER
1 HANDFUL (OR MORE) ORGANIC LEAFY GREENS
2 PIECES (OR MORE) ORGANIC FRUIT
1 HANDFUL ICE (OPTIONAL)

In a blender, combine the water, greens, fruit, and ice. Blend until smooth. Serve immediately.

VARIATIONS

Herbs: Herbs are full of nutrition and pack tons of flavor. Make a green smoothie with fresh herbs added, like oregano, rosemary, basil, and dill.

Organic edible flowers: These make a lovely addition to a smoothie, and they also pack some fabulous nutrition. In some recipes, they'll add noticeable little flecks of pretty colors. Pre-packed assortments of organic edible flowers are often available next to the fresh herbs in the produce section of natural foods stores.

Stevia: Stevia is a great sweetener option for green smoothies when you want to use less fruit. Fresh stevia leaves are best, but if you don't have any available, you can find stevia in your local natural foods store. It's available in liquid, white powder, or green powder form. If I can't get it fresh, I try to buy the green powder version because it's the least processed of the options. My favorite brand is Navitas Naturals.

Extracts and flavorings: Add ½ to 1 teaspoon of raw vanilla powder (or any flavor extract) or ground cinnamon, nutmeg, or other spice to make your smoothie more interesting and fun.

GARAM MASALA GREEN SMOOTHIE

MAKES 1 TO 2 SERVINGS

This delicious smoothie is hydrating and nourishing, with the perfect amount of light sweetness. I particularly enjoy it as a breakfast smoothie that is great on the go.

2 CUPS (400 G) PEELED AND CHOPPED BANANA
1 CUP (240 ML) RAW ALMOND MILK (PAGE 177)
1 CUP (30 G) PACKED SPINACH
1 CUP (130 G) CHOPPED CUCUMBER
1 HANDFUL ICE
2 TABLESPOONS CHIA SEEDS
1 TEASPOON GARAM MASALA

In a blender, combine the banana, almond milk, spinach, cucumber, ice, chia seeds, and garam masala. Blend until smooth. Serve immediately.

PURPLE PASSION SMOOTHIE

MAKES 4 CUPS (950 ML)

This is a popular smoothie that is chock-full of nutrition. I love making it with oranges picked right off the tree in my mom's backyard. Mmmm! Although it's purple in color, it classifies as a green smoothie, because of the spinach.

1½ CUPS (360 ML) WATER
1½ CUPS (225 G) FROZEN BLUEBERRIES
1½ CUPS (340 G) ORANGE SEGMENTS
1½ CUPS (45 G) PACKED SPINACH LEAVES
DASH OF STEVIA (OPTIONAL)

In a blender, combine the water, blueberries, orange, spinach, and stevia (if using). Blend until smooth. Serve immediately.

ORANGE-VANILLA CREAM PROTEIN SMOOTHIE

MAKES 1 TO 2 SERVINGS

This is a fabulous smoothie that reminds me of a Creamsicle. Another way to enjoy it, equally as delish but different, is with ½ teaspoon of ground cinnamon added.

1 CUP (240 ML) RAW ALMOND MILK (PAGE 177)
1 HANDFUL ICE
1 CUP (200 G) CHOPPED BANANA
¾ CUP (175 ML) FRESH ORANGE JUICE
3 TABLESPOONS HEMP PROTEIN POWDER
1 TABLESPOON FLAX MEAL
½ TEASPOON RAW VANILLA POWDER
GRATED ZEST OF 1 ORANGE

In a blender, combine the almond milk, ice, banana, orange juice, protein powder, flax meal, vanilla powder, and orange zest. Blend until smooth. Serve immediately.

VANILLA-BLACKBERRY FROSTY

MAKES 1 SERVING

This drink can be served for breakfast, snack, or dessert (which is often the case with raw foods, because they're so versatile!). Its vibrant color is gorgeous, and using almond milk as the base gives your body magnesium, manganese, vitamin E, and many other nutrients.

1 CUP (240 ML) RAW ALMOND MILK (PAGE 177)
1 CUP (140 G) FROZEN BLACKBERRIES
2 TO 3 TEASPOONS RAW AGAVE NECTAR
¼ TEASPOON RAW VANILLA POWDER

In a blender, combine the almond milk, blackberries, agave nectar, and vanilla powder. Blend until smooth. Serve immediately.

CHOCOLATE CRUNCH FROSTY

MAKES 2 SERVINGS

I make this frosty a lot, and I mean a lot! My husband's face lights up every time I bring one to him. The cacao nibs add a delightful crunch with every slurp. (I'm a texture girl, so I love crunchy with my creamy.)

2¼ CUPS (540 ML) RAW ALMOND MILK (PAGE 177)
3 FROZEN BANANAS, CHOPPED
3 TABLESPOONS RAW CHOCOLATE POWDER
2 TABLESPOONS RAW CACAO NIBS
½ TEASPOON CHOCOLATE EXTRACT

In a blender, combine the almond milk, bananas, chocolate powder, cacao nibs, and chocolate extract. Blend until smooth. Serve immediately.

CUCUMBER-CARROT JUICE

MAKES 1 TO 2 SERVINGS

Cucumbers and carrots are wonderful for your skin. If you want a gorgeous glow, you need to feed yourself right. Start with this juice!

2 LARGE CUCUMBERS
2 LARGE CARROTS

Using a juicer, juice the cucumbers and carrots. Serve immediately.

ITALIAN POWER JUICE

MAKES 2 SERVINGS

Here's a great way to start your day! Power Juice will jump start your day with alkalizing and immune-boosting ingredients that taste great and make you feel great.

2 MEDIUM TO LARGE CUCUMBERS

½ BUNCH CELERY

1 SMALL TO MEDIUM FENNEL BULB, TRIMMED (NO STALKS)

3 PLUM (ROMA) TOMATOES

1 GARLIC CLOVE

4 LARGE SWISS CHARD LEAVES

Using your juicer, juice the cucumbers, celery, fennel bulb, tomatoes, garlic, and Swiss chard. Serve immediately.

KALE KIWI IMMUNE-BOOSTING JUICE

MAKES 2 SERVINGS

If you're looking for a juice to help you get over a cold or flu, here it is. Kiwifruit is loaded with vitamin C, and cucumbers are über-hydrating. And, kale? Too many kick-ass nutrients to name here.

1 BUNCH PURPLE KALE

1 BUNCH CELERY

2 LARGE CUCUMBERS

2 KIWIS

Using a juicer, juice the kale, celery, cucumbers, and kiwis. Serve immediately.

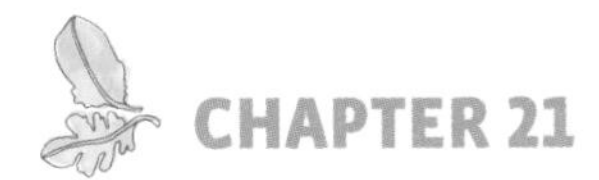

CHAPTER 21

DESSERTS

STRAWBERRY SOFT SERVE

MAKES 1 TO 2 SERVINGS

Having soft serve this creamy and delicious should be sinful, but . . . it's not! It's wonderfully healthful, fun, and perfect any time of the day.

¾ CUP (180 ML) RAW ALMOND MILK (PAGE 177)
1 CUP (150 G) FROZEN STRAWBERRIES OR ANY FROZEN BERRIES
STEVIA OR RAW AGAVE NECTAR

In a blender, combine the almond milk and berries. Blend to a soft-serve ice cream texture. Sweeten to taste with stevia and serve immediately.

CHOCOLATE-BANANA VELVET ICE CREAM

MAKES 4 SERVINGS

Having a ready-to-use supply of frozen bananas in your freezer is a must! The best way to do this is by peeling ripe bananas and using a FoodSaver for storage. This ensures they don't get ice crystals on them and helps maintain their nutrition and color. If you don't have a FoodSaver yet, put the peeled bananas in a baggie (or other container) in the freezer.

4 FROZEN BANANAS, CHOPPED AND THAWED SLIGHTLY
¼ CUP (30 G) RAW CHOCOLATE POWDER
2 TABLESPOONS RAW AGAVE NECTAR
¼ CUP (60 ML) WATER

In a blender or food processor, combine the bananas, chocolate powder, agave nectar, and water. Process until smooth. Serve immediately.

CHOCOLATE-MINT ICY

MAKES 2 SERVINGS

Chocolate and mint are my favorite flavors to combine. This particular recipe is extra good because the ice takes it to a whole new level. Want a refreshing dessert or snack for warmer weather? This will do the trick.

½ CUP (55 G) RAW CASHEWS
½ CUP (7 G) FRESH MINT LEAVES
3 TABLESPOONS RAW AGAVE NECTAR
2 HANDFULS ICE
1 CUP (240 ML) WATER
¼ CUP (30 G) RAW CHOCOLATE POWDER
PINCH OF HIMALAYAN CRYSTAL SALT

Put the cashews in a bowl and add water to cover by about 1 inch (2.5 cm). Let the cashews soak at room temperature for 1 to 2 hours.

Drain the cashews, rinse them, and put in a blender. Add the mint, agave nectar, ice, water, chocolate powder, and salt. Blend until relatively smooth. Serve immediately.

SWEET CHIA PUDDING

MAKES 2 SERVINGS

Chia pudding is a great dessert that is loaded with nutrition from the essential fatty acids, calcium, and more. Plus, it's easy and fun to make.

¼ CUP (35 G) CHIA SEEDS
1 CUP (240 ML) RAW ALMOND MILK (PAGE 177)
2 TO 3 TABLESPOONS RAW AGAVE NECTAR
DASH OF ALMOND EXTRACT OR VANILLA EXTRACT

Put the chia seeds in a small bowl. Blend the almond milk with the agave nectar and almond extract in a blender. Pour the liquid into the bowl with the chia seeds. Stir the mixture. Wait a few minutes, then stir and wait two more times. The mixture will congeal. Eat now or refrigerate until chilled.

VARIATION: I also like making this with raw Brazil nut milk or raw cashew milk.

VANILLA CHAI PEACH COBBLER

MAKES ONE 8-INCH- (20-CM-) SQUARE COBBLER

Raw cobblers are a stealthy way to sneak delicious raw ingredients into your family's diet. They're impossible to turn down once someone has had a taste, and this recipe, in particular, is a real star. My husband begs me to make it every couple of weeks. If you warm this in a dehydrator, it intensifies the flavors beautifully.

CRUMBLE

2 CUPS (230 G) RAW PECANS

1/2 CUP (40 G) UNSWEETENED SHREDDED COCONUT

1/4 TEASPOON HIMALAYAN CRYSTAL SALT

3/4 CUP (130 G) RAISINS

VANILLA CHAI PEACH FILLING

THREE 10-OUNCE (284-G) BAGS FROZEN PEACHES, THAWED

10 MEDJOOL DATES, PITTED

4 WHOLE CLOVES

1 TEASPOON RAW VANILLA POWDER

3/4 TEASPOON GROUND CINNAMON

3/4 TEASPOON GINGER POWDER

1/2 TEASPOON GROUND CARDAMOM

1/2 TEASPOON GROUND ALLSPICE

PINCH OF GROUND BLACK PEPPER

FOR THE CRUMBLE: In a food processor, combine the pecans, coconut, and salt. Process until coarsely ground. Add the raisins and process until the mixture resembles coarse crumbs and holds together when gently pressed between two fingers. Set aside.

FOR THE FILLING: Chop one bag of peaches. Put the chopped peaches in a large bowl and set aside. In a blender, combine the remaining two bags of peaches with the dates, cloves, vanilla powder, cinnamon, ginger powder, cardamom, allspice, and pepper. Blend until smooth. Pour the blended mixture into the bowl with the chopped peaches and stir well.

Pour half of the crumble into the bottom of an 8-inch (20-cm or 2-L) square baking dish and give it a firm but gentle press. Spread the peach filling on top. Sprinkle the remaining crumble on top of the peach filling. Serve at room temperature, or warm in a dehydrator for up to 2 hours at 130°F (54°C).

CITRUS-ALMOND CHEESECAKE

MAKES ONE 8-INCH (20-CM) CAKE

Raw cheesecakes are a great dessert for impressing friends and family. But you can also make one for just yourself! Slice it after it sets and freeze the individual slices. Then, take a slice out to thaw when you want a heavenly dessert. Bonus: This cheesecake is really easy to make.

CRUST

2 CUPS (230 G) RAW WALNUTS OR RAW PECANS
1/2 CUP (85 G) RAISINS, GENTLY PACKED
GRATED ZEST OF 1 ORANGE
GRATED ZEST OF 1/2 LIME

FILLING

3 CUPS (345 G) RAW CASHEWS
3/4 CUP (180 ML) RAW AGAVE NECTAR
1/4 CUP (60 ML) FRESH ORANGE JUICE
1/4 CUP (60 ML) FRESH LIME JUICE
1 TABLESPOON ALMOND EXTRACT
GRATED ZEST OF 1 ORANGE
GRATED ZEST OF 1/2 LIME
1/8 TEASPOON HIMALAYAN CRYSTAL SALT
2/3 CUP (160 ML) COCONUT OIL
2 TABLESPOONS SOY LECITHIN (NON-GMO); SEE NOTE

FOR THE CRUST: In a food processor, grind the nuts until coarsely ground. Add the raisins, orange zest, and lime zest and process until the mixture begins to gently stick together when pressed between two of your fingers. Press the crust mixture firmly into the bottom of an 8-inch (20-cm) springform pan. Set aside.

FOR THE FILLING: Put the cashews in a bowl and add water to cover by about 1 inch (2.5 cm). Let the cashews soak at room temperature for 1 to 2 hours. Drain and give them a quick rinse. Add the nuts and the agave nectar, orange juice, lime juice, almond extract, orange zest, lime zest, salt, and coconut oil to the food processor and process until creamy (3 to 5 minutes). You may need to stop every couple of minutes to scrape down the sides of the processor. Add the soy lecithin and process to incorporate.

Pour the filling over the crust and smooth with an offset spatula. Refrigerate or freeze for a few hours, or until set. Serve or cover and store in refrigerator for up to 1 week.

NOTE: Soy lecithin is not raw but is recommended to achieve a firmer texture.

DATE BARS

MAKES 12 TO 16 BARS

When I was a little girl, my mom used to make date bars for dessert. Oh, how I loved them! She used a mix from a box (Betty Crocker, I think). The bars were warm from the oven with a sweet, squishy date center and a crumbly bottom and top. Mmmm! So, I decided to come up with a healthier raw version. This one is warm from the dehydrator with a squishy, sweet raw date filling with a slightly crunchy top and bottom from ground nuts (but if you don't have a dehydrator, no worries! Make them anyway.). When I shared them with my mom, she couldn't believe how closely they resembled the old version.

27 MEDJOOL DATES, PITTED

CRUMBLE

1 CUP (115 G) RAW ALMONDS
1 CUP (115 G) RAW CASHEWS
¼ CUP (35 G) RAW COCONUT CRYSTALS
2 TABLESPOONS RAW COCONUT OIL
PINCH OF HIMALAYAN CRYSTAL SALT

Put the dates in a bowl and add water to cover. Soak them for 20 to 30 minutes. Drain, reserving ¼ cup (60 ml) of the water. Put the dates in a food processor with the reserved soaking water. Process until smooth. Set aside in a bowl while you make the crumble.

FOR THE CRUMBLE: In a food processor, combine the almonds, cashews, coconut crystals, coconut oil, and salt. Process until the mixture starts to stick together a bit when pressed gently between your fingers.

Take about two-thirds of the crumble mixture and press it firmly into the bottom of an 8x8-inch (20x20-cm or 2-L) glass baking dish. Gently spread the date filling on top. Sprinkle the remaining crumble on top of the date filling and gently press it with your hand.

If you have a dehydrator, put the baking dish on a dehydrator tray and dehydrate the bars at 125°F (52°C) for about 1 hour, or until warm. Store leftover bars in your refrigerator for up to 5 days.

FIVE-MINUTE WALNUT-OATMEAL BROWNIES

MAKES 12 TO 16 BROWNIES

These are especially great because the oats help keep the calorie count low without sacrificing flavor.

1 CUP (115 G) WALNUTS
1 CUP (85 G) RAW OATS
3/4 CUP (80 G) RAW CHOCOLATE POWDER
22 SOFT MEDJOOL DATES, PITTED (SEE NOTE)
3/4 TEASPOON ALMOND EXTRACT

In a food processor, grind the walnuts until coarsely ground. Add the oats and chocolate powder and process until thoroughly mixed. Add the dates and almond extract and process until the mixture holds together when gently pressed between two of your fingers. Transfer the mixture to an 8-inch (20-cm or 2-L) square glass baking dish and press it in firmly. Serve at room temperature, or warm in a dehydrator for up to 2 hours at 130°F (54°C).

NOTE: If your Medjool dates are on the small side, you might want to add a few more to the recipe. Medjool dates from BlueMountain Organics.com are big, plump, and soft.

RAW FOOD GLOSSARY

Here's a list of popular ingredients used in raw food. For those that can't be purchased at your local health food store, I've included online resources.

BANANAS (FROZEN)

To make frozen bananas, simply peel ripe bananas, place them in a baggie or container, and put them in the freezer. I like to use my FoodSaver, because it keeps the bananas from getting ice crystals on them. Having frozen bananas in your freezer at all times is a smart move. They are fantastic in smoothies, and they make a deliciously fun raw ice cream (just throw them in the food processor and puree them into a soft-serve, raw vegan ice cream).

BREAD (SPROUTED)

Available at natural foods stores. A couple of my favorite brands are Good for Life and Manna Organics. These are not raw but they are the healthiest cooked breads that I know of.

CACAO LIQUOR (RAW)

Whole cacao beans that have been peeled and cold-pressed into a paste. It is used to make a number of raw chocolate recipes. It comes in a block form and can be melted into a thick liquid in a dehydrator or double boiler. It's bitter, so I add sweetener. Available from NavitasNaturals.com.

CACAO NIBS (RAW)

Partially ground cacao beans that can be used in a variety of ways, from toppings to raw vegan ice cream or yogurt. They add texture to shakes and smoothies, and you can make raw chocolates with them. They are available from NavitasNaturals.com and other sources online.

CAROB (RAW)

A lot of the carob you find in the store is toasted (so look for the word "raw" on the label). I like to use raw carob, which has a wonderful caramel-like flavor and can be used in many recipes such as smoothies, nut milks, desserts, and more. There is a link for raw carob at KristensRaw.com/store.

CHIA SEEDS

Known as the "dieter's dream food," chia seeds are praised for many things, including their fantastic nutrient profile, which proudly boasts iron, boron, essential fatty acids, fiber, and more. Add to that the claims that they may improve heart health, reduce blood pressure, stabilize blood sugar, and help people lose weight by giving them extra stamina and energy and curbing hunger, and you might become a fan of these little guys, too. They're superstars in my book. You can find a link for them at KristensRaw.com/store.

CHOCOLATE (CACAO) POWDER (RAW)

Made from cacao beans that have been peeled and cold-pressed. Then, the cacao oil is extracted, leaving a powder. Use in many recipes, from raw chocolate desserts to smoothies to soups to dressings and more. Available from NavitasNaturals.com and other sources online.

COCONUT AMINOS

A seasoning sauce that can be used in place of tamari and namo shoyu. Available from CoconutSecret.com and Whole Foods Markets, it's raw, enzymatically alive, organic, gluten-free, and soy-free.

COCONUT BUTTER OR SPREAD (RAW)

Not to be confused with plain coconut oil, coconut butter is a mixture of coconut oil and coconut meat. It can be eaten by the spoonful and be used in desserts, smoothies, spreads, and more. Available from WildernessFamilyNaturals.com as coconut spread, and from Artisana as coconut butter. Artisana coconut butter is available at many natural foods stores, including Whole Foods Market. To make coconut butter softer and easier to use, warm it in a dehydrator at a low temperature.

DIAYA CHEESE

This is an amazing vegan cheese (not raw) that is taking the vegan world by storm. If you know of people who miss artery-clogging, animal-based cheese, then turn them on to this amazing product made from—get this—tapioca! It's soy-free, dairy-free, gluten-free, corn-free, and preservative-free. See more details at DaiyaFoods.com. Available at Whole Foods Market.

GOJI BERRIES

These little ruby-colored jewels (also known as wolfberries) are a mega-popular superfood because of their amazing nutrient content. They have eighteen amino acids, including the eight essential amino acids. Plus, their antioxidants are through the roof! The taste is a cross between a dried cherry and dried cranberry. Enjoy them plain and in various recipes. Available from NavitasNaturals.com and in many natural foods stores; see a link at KristensRaw.com/store.

GOLDEN BERRIES

Also known as Incan berries or Cape gooseberries, these are dried fruits similar in shape to a raisin and golden in color. Golden berries will throw a party in your mouth. They are available at NavitasNaturals.com.

GREEN POWDER(S)

Made from dark greens and other vegetables, these are chock-full of powerful raw and alkalizing nutrition. My favorites are Health Force Nutritionals' Vitamineral Green and Amazing Grass' Wheat Grass Powder. Health Force Nutritionals also makes a green powder for pets called Green Mush. You will find links to these products at KristensRaw.com/store.

HEMP FOODS

Hemp is commonly referred to as a "superfood" because of its amazing nutritional value. Its amino acid profile dominates, with the eight essential amino acids (ten if you're elderly or a baby), making it a vegan source of "complete" protein. Manitoba Harvest is my favorite source for hemp products. You can use their hemp seeds, hemp butter, hemp protein powder, and hemp oil to make many delicious raw foods.

HERBAMERE

This blend of sea salt and fourteen organic herbs is a nice change of pace from plain salt. Available from Amazon.com, other Web sites, and some natural foods stores.

LUCUMA POWDER

A fun ingredient made from a Peruvian fruit that is popular with raw fooders. Available from NavitasNaturals.com and other online sources, lucuma is a whole-food powder that adds a lovely sweetness to recipes and has a flavor that has been described as a cross between sweet potato and maple. Use lucuma powder in various raw recipes for smoothies, ice cream, cheesecake, nut milk, cookies, brownies, and more.

MACA POWDER

Made from a plant used as a medicinal herb, this powder is said to give users stamina, tons of energy, and an increased libido! I'm not a huge fan of maca's pungent flavor, but it is a popular superfood among raw vegans. There is a link for maca powder at KristensRaw.com/store.

MESQUITE POWDER

A nutritional powder with a smoky, malt-like caramel flavor, made from pods of the mesquite tree. Available from NavitasNaturals.com and other online sources.

MISO

Miso is a protein seasoning known for its role in Japanese cuisine. It's usually made from a combination of soybeans, cultured grain, and sea salt by a fermentation process. Miso contains all of the essential amino acids, making it a complete protein. Miso is not raw, but due to the presence of beneficial digestive enzymes, unpasteurized miso is considered to be a "living food." South River Miso makes the best organic miso. They have so many amazing flavors (including soy-free varieties). Check them out at SouthRiverMiso.com.

MULBERRIES

Lightly sweet, with a wonderful texture that makes it hard to stop eating them, these delights have great nutrient content and are a decent source of protein. Available in dry form from NavitasNaturals.com.

NONDAIRY (PLANT-BASED) MILK

Many plant-based milks are available for purchase in various grocery stores. They are not raw, but they are vegan and many are organic, which I highly recommend. Options include almond, hemp, rice, soy, hazelnut, oat, and coconut. Plus, there are different flavors within those varieties, such as vanilla and chocolate.

NUT/SEED BUTTERS (RAW)

Raw nut butters can be bought at most natural foods stores, or you can easily make your own (simply grind nuts with a dash of Himalayan crystal salt in a food processor until a paste forms). You might choose to add a little olive oil to help facilitate the processing. Different varieties include hemp seed, almond, hazelnut, pecan, sunflower seed, pumpkin seed, cashew, walnut, macadamia nut, and more. Some excellent brands are Living Tree Community, Rejuvenative Brands, Wilderness Poets (online), and Artisana. Many are available from Whole Foods Market.

OLIVES (RAW)

Essential Living Foods' black bojita olives are juicy, fresh, and delicious. Available at Whole Foods Market and online at EssentialLivingFoods.com. I also use Living Tree Community's Sun-Dried Olives in some recipes.

OLIVE OIL (RAW)

Not all cold-pressed olive oils are raw. Two truly raw brands are Living Tree Community (available at LivingTreeCommunity.com and some Whole Foods Markets) and Wilderness Family Naturals (available online at Wilderness FamilyNaturals.com).

PROTEIN POWDER

Add extra protein to your diet with protein shakes made from vegan protein powders. My favorites are hemp sprouted raw brown rice powders. Try Sprout Living's EPIC Protein or the chocolate and natural flavors from Sun Warrior. Available at KristensRaw.com/store.

RAPADURA

This is a dried sugarcane juice, and it's not raw. It is, however, an unrefined and unbleached organic whole-cane sugar. Available at Whole Foods Market.

RIGHTEOUSLY RAW CACAO BARS

This organic, raw, vegan chocolate bar is the best raw chocolate bar on the market. My favorite flavor is the caramel cacao, but Earch Choice Organics also sells goji, maca, and acai. Sometimes I just don't have time to make my own raw chocolate, and sometimes I'm just plain lazy. In both cases, I run to Whole Foods Market for these (you can also buy them online direct from the company: EarthSourceOrganics.com). If your Whole Foods doesn't stock these . . . tell them to do it! Check out my blog post where I talked about my first encounter with these divine treats, KristensRaw.blogspot.com/2010/03/review-earth-source-organics.html.

ROLLED OATS

Raw oats (processed with special cold-rolling machinery designed to preserve nutritional value) are available at NaturalZing.com.

SAUERKRAUT (RAW, UNPASTEURIZED)

You can buy sauerkraut from the natural foods store or make it yourself (my favorite way). If you choose to buy it from the store, be sure to get a brand that is organic, raw, and unpasteurized. Two brands I like are Gold Mine Natural Foods and Rejuvenative Foods (they're both great, but my overall preference is Gold Mine Natural Foods). However, making your own is the best. It's incredibly easy and fun. For directions on making your own sauerkraut, please see my blog posts and video at KristensRaw.blogspot.com/2009/07/how-to-make-sauerkraut-video-raw.html.

SESAME OIL (RAW)

Most sesame oils you find in health food stores are made from toasted sesame. You can get raw sesame oil from RejuvenativeFoods.com.

STEVIA

An all-natural sweetener, made from the leaves of the stevia plant, that does not elevate blood sugar levels. It is very sweet, so you will want to use much less stevia than you would any other sweetener. A truly raw, green-colored variety is available from NavitasNaturals.com. (Stevia you find in stores is usually processed, not raw, and white in color or liquid.)

SUN-DRIED OLIVES

Look for the Living Tree Community at Whole Foods Market or online at LivingTreeCommunity.com.

SUNFLOWER LECITHIN

Popular for its choline content, lecithin is also used as an emulsifier in recipes. Soy lecithin is a common source for this purpose, but not everyone wants a soy product. That has all changed now that sunflower lecithin is available. Add it to raw soups, smoothies, desserts, and more. You can find a link for it at KristensRaw.com/store.

TEECCINO

A non-raw alkaline herbal "coffee" made from barley and chicory. Available at many natural foods stores and online at Amazon.com. For details about the awesomeness of this delicious coffee substitute, check out Teeccino.com.

WAKAME FLAKES

Available from NavitasNaturals.com and many natural foods stores, wakame is a sea vegetable that contains essential minerals, antioxidants, omega-3 fatty acids, vitamins C and B complex, and fiber. This is a great way to add flavor and nutrition to salads, dressings, and soups.

WHEATGRASS POWDER

Look for Amazing Grass' Wheat Grass Powder, available at KristensRaw.com/store. Add it to smoothies and juices, or just drink it down with water to add a huge nutritional punch every day.

YACÓN SYRUP, POWDER, AND SLICES

Made from a Peruvian Andes root, Yacón is an alternative sweetener with a low glycemic index. Available from NavitasNaturals.com.

INDEX